D1477077

# National Guidelines
## for the Use of Complementary Therapies in Supportive and Palliative Care

## Marianne Tavares

The Prince of Wales's Foundation for Integrated Health

The National Council for Hospice and Specialist Palliative Care Services

Supported by Lloyds TSB Foundation for England and Wales

The Prince of Wales's Foundation for Integrated Health
London, England

National Guidelines for the Use of Complementary Therapies in Supportive and Palliative Care by Marianne Tavares

ISBN 0 9539453 5 9

The Prince of Wales's Foundation for Integrated Health
12 Chillingworth Road
London N7 8QJ
020 7619 6140

www.fihealth.org.uk
email: info@fihealth.org.uk

Disclaimer

# Foreword

## by HRH The Prince of Wales

I am delighted to have the opportunity of introducing these National Guidelines for the Use of Complementary Therapies in Supportive and Palliative Care which have been developed by my Foundation for Integrated Health working in partnership with the National Council for Hospice and Specialist Palliative Care Services.

Complementary therapies are becoming increasingly available to patients suffering from long-term or chronic illness as an integral part of the palliative and supportive care that they receive in hospital wards, hospices, cancer support centres and at home. These guidelines will, I am sure, prove to be invaluable to managers and providers of these services and will, hopefully, give them the confidence to extend the range of therapies that they provide. They are clear, concise and comprehensive and will go a long way towards ensuring that complementary therapies are delivered safely, effectively and appropriately and in a way that will bring the most benefit to patients.

Patients are increasingly demanding a more holistic approach to their treatment; an approach which takes into account their physical, mental and spiritual wellbeing. I look forward to the day when these healing therapies will become available to all those who would benefit from them and I very much hope that these excellent guidelines will help carry this process forward.

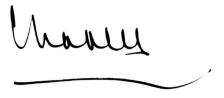

# Preface

by Professor Mike Richards,
National Cancer Director

A substantial number of cancer patients choose to receive complementary therapies alongside their mainstream cancer treatment. Individual patients frequently report that the use of a complementary therapy has helped them. Despite this, it has been difficult to generate convincing research evidence of the benefits of these therapies with respect to the amelioration of physical or psychological symptoms. Because of this, decision making regarding the provision of complementary therapy services remains complex both for commissioners and service providers.

There is broad agreement, however, that patients should have ready access to reliable information about complementary therapies and complementary therapy services. It is also important that where services are provided this is done in a way which protects patients' safety.

These guidelines address issues which are directly related to patient safety in the provision of complementary therapy services, including clinical governance, regulation and training of therapists and audit and evaluation. The guidelines will usefully complement the forthcoming NICE guidance on supportive and palliative care.

Professor M A Richards

May 2003

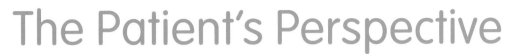

# The Patient's Perspective

Why use complementary therapies in supportive and palliative care?

" For oft, when on my couch I lie
    In vacant or in pensive mood,
    They flash upon that inward eye
    Which is the bliss of solitude…"
William Wordsworth (1770 – 1850)

"Marion's massages were something to look forward to, something nice that happened in the daily round of unpleasantness. I was more able to accept what was happening to me, more ready to deal with the treatment, simply was in a better frame of mind to heal myself."
(Izod 1996)

"It has meant that I no longer get tummy cramps and awful wind. I am able to go to the toilet once a day instead of feeling that I need to go several times a day."
(Preece 2002)

"I am now sleeping through the night."
"Headaches are almost gone or are coped with."
"My energy levels are increased."
(Wright et al 2002)

"When the healing started I began to calm a little. I realised this was my time to receive… and that I was beginning to connect with my inner feelings and acknowledge my emotions.  After approximately four sessions I began to feel huge surges of energy, a high following the healing. My healer made sure that I was grounded before I left and I learnt to direct and use this energy myself and to call upon it when I needed it."
(Penson 1998)

"It was wonderful, I completely forgot about everything that was being done to my body, and got lost in the gentle music and massage."

"I felt very good, the pain seemed to go out of my body. Massage did definitely help very much."
(Corner et al 1995)

# Contents

# 1 Executive Summary

1.1 These guidelines bring together the different issues and questions that organisations face when considering the development of complementary therapy services in supportive and palliative care. The guidelines have been written for the use of managers and those responsible for developing complementary therapy services in both the statutory and voluntary sectors, and for self-help groups. The focus is mainly on cancer, although information is also given about key clinical issues for people with motor neurone disease, Parkinson's disease and multiple sclerosis.

1.2 The term complementary therapies refers to those therapies which are used alongside conventional health care. Surveys show that over 30% of people with cancer use complementary therapies (Rees et al 2000, Lewith et al 2002). Most provision is in hospices (36%) and hospitals (31%), with up to 20% based in the voluntary sector (Kohn 2003). The touch therapies, such as aromatherapy, massage and reflexology, are provided in over 90% of services; mind-body therapies, for example relaxation and visualisation, in over 80% and healing and energy work by about 45% of service providers (Kohn 2003).

1.3 The guidelines set out a range of issues to be considered when developing services; these come under two main headings:
- service development and management
- practice development

Service development includes clinical governance, the regulation and training of therapists, recruitment and selection, and the management of volunteer therapists. Practice development considers professional and ethical issues, supervision, clinical issues, referral and assessment, and the use of nine therapies.

The guidelines provide additional advice for practitioners on ethical issues, which include:
- the importance of respecting the patient's choice in all areas of their care
- the need for professionals to recognise and respect the role and contribution of conventional health care colleagues within supportive and palliative care
- the importance of not making any claims for complementary therapy treatments

1.4 The nine therapies included are the touch therapies of aromatherapy, massage and reflexology; the healing and energy therapies of reiki, spiritual healing and therapeutic touch; hypnosis and hypnotherapy; acupuncture; and homeopathy. For each, the best available evidence is reviewed, and information is given about the conditions for which each therapy may be useful. Guidance is also given on contraindications and precautions for the use of these therapies in supportive and palliative care.

1.5 The guidelines provide an outline of the current situation regarding the regulation, training and qualifications of therapists and gives useful information about recruiting therapists. In addition, guidance is given on the position and recruitment of volunteer therapists.

1.6 Broad advice is given in relation to clinical governance and the development of complementary therapy services. Suggestions are made for the different ways in which clinical governance could be implemented.

1.7 A wide range of other complementary therapies are used in supportive and palliative care, and it has not proved possible to include detailed information about all of them. Useful contact information is given in the appendices. The Macmillan Directory (2002) also provides valuable information on organisations which offer therapies not included in these guidelines.

# 2 Introduction

## 2.1 Background

These guidelines bring together the different issues and questions that organisations face when considering the development of complementary therapy services in supportive and palliative care. This introduction explains the need for national guidelines, outlines the scope of the guidelines and gives definitions for supportive and palliative care.

The use of complementary therapies following a diagnosis of cancer is a significant and growing phenomenon. One recent survey of 1023 women with breast cancer showed that 31.5% had consulted a complementary therapist since diagnosis (Rees et al 2000). Another survey showed that 32% (n=162) of those with cancer were receiving complementary therapy treatments, whilst 49% of those not receiving them would like to have complementary therapy treatments (Lewith et al 2002).

A survey of the provision of complementary therapies, conducted in 108 hospice and palliative care units, showed that the most popular therapies were massage (76 units), aromatherapy (73 units), and relaxation (71 units). (Wilkes 1992) Research on access to complementary medicine via general practice (Thomas et al 2001) indicated that 39.5% of general practice partnerships in England provided access to some form of complementary therapy for their national health service patients.

*The Directory of Complementary Therapy Services in UK Cancer Care* produced by Macmillan Cancer Relief (Macmillan 2002) shows widespread use of complementary therapies in the UK. Most provision is in hospices (36%) and hospitals (31%), with up to 20% based in the voluntary sector (Kohn 2003). Of the 40 or more therapies offered (Macmillan 2002) those most commonly provided are the touch therapies, such as aromatherapy, massage and reflexology, in over 90% of services, and mind-body therapies, for instance relaxation and visualisation, in over 80% of services (Kohn 2003). Healing and energy work including reiki, spiritual healing and therapeutic touch, are also widely available in 45% of services.

The impetus to develop national guidelines came from the National Council for Hospice and Specialist Palliative Care Services and The Prince of Wales's Foundation for Integrated Health. The project was funded by The Lloyds TSB Foundation for England and Wales.

In October 2001, a request was made to about 500 providers of supportive and palliative care in the UK,

as listed in the *2001 Directory of Hospice and Palliative Care Services*, for local guidelines, policies, standards and protocols. Approximately 100 sets of policies or standards (20%) were received, and about another 20 organisations replied that policies were being developed or reviewed. It is not known whether this response rate is an indication of lack of policies despite the widespread use of complementary therapies shown in the Macmillan directory. It is known, however, that there are an increasing number of enquiries to the National Association of Complementary Therapists in Hospice and Palliative Care for guidance on the development of policies.

## 2.2 The need for national guidelines

### Clinical governance

While the framework of clinical governance (Department of Health 1999) applies to NHS organisations, it is becoming equally important for services in the voluntary sector to be able to demonstrate to funders their determination to safeguard quality of care. Complementary therapy services are not exempt from the same scrutiny. Indeed, the process of safeguarding quality of care within complementary therapy services is likely to inspire confidence and encourage integration with conventional health care, as recommended by the House of Lords Report on complementary and alternative medicine (House of Lords 2000). The purpose of these national guidelines is to provide information and recommend activities which can contribute to quality improvement, patient safety and improved outcomes.

### NICE guidance on supportive and palliative care

Complementary therapies will be included as one aspect of the forthcoming *Guidance on Improving Supportive and Palliative Care for Adults with Cancer*, which is being developed under the auspices of the National Institute for Clinical Excellence (NICE), and commissioned by the Department of Health. The purpose of the NICE guidance is to identify service models most likely to lead to high quality care for people with cancer and their carers and it will make a series of recommendations about service provision, planning and workforce development. It is due to be published towards the end of 2003.

These guidelines for the use of complementary therapies in supportive and palliative care consider a broader range of issues within service development, for example recruitment, qualifications and training, supervision, referral and assessment. Also included is a review of the evidence base for the use of the key therapies in supportive and palliative care.

Evidence

The focus of the government's 10 year programme to improve the NHS, as set out in the white paper, *The new NHS, modern, dependable* (DoH 1997), is primarily on evidence-based integrated care, quality assurance, clinical and cost effectiveness, and performance management. Commissioners and service providers call for evidence to support the use of complementary therapies in palliative care. The factors which have hindered research into the effectiveness of complementary therapies are well-documented (Penson 1998, Dunn et al 1995; Hobbs & Davies 1998), as are the difficulties of conducting research with people with a life-threatening condition or advanced and progressive illness (Donnelly 2000, Karim 2000).

The emerging picture shows that the evidence base is greater for some therapies than others. Professionals with a conventional medical or scientific background believe that in order for complementary therapies to be more widely accepted, it is important "that they have a critical mass of scientifically-controlled evidence to support their claims and that at the moment most therapies lack such evidence" (House of Lords 2000). Following the House of Lords report and the government's response, a framework for increasing research capacity in complementary and alternative medicine is currently being developed by the Department of Health (see www.doh.gov.uk/research). There is a need for more research from a variety of perspectives and methodological approaches.

However, lack of evidence is not necessarily evidence of a lack of effectiveness. It is clear from numerous surveys and service evaluations that patients value the use of complementary therapies as an integral part of their care. It may be useful to remember that evidence based practice has been described as the conscientious, explicit, and judicious use of current best evidence in making decisions about the care of individual patients (Sackett 1996). Evidence based practice requires practitioners to integrate the best external evidence with individual clinical expertise and the patient's choice (Sackett 1996).

These guidelines have been written, based on the best available evidence, to facilitate the development of services and to encourage the integration of complementary therapy services in supportive and palliative care. Although such services are provided in a large and growing number of organisations, provision remains patchy and without equality of access.

Regulation

The Prince of Wales's Foundation for Integrated Health is working with eighteen different therapies who are working towards more robust regulation, statutory or voluntary. However, the groups are currently at different stages of development, which means that standards of practice may vary, and patients may be exposed to inconsistent, inappropriate or even poor quality care. Although many excellent models of practice exist, the lack of consensus on standards not only causes confusion for patients when considering a therapy or therapist, but also raises issues for health care providers when it comes to recruitment. For example, what constitutes acceptable qualifications and registration requirements for the different therapies, and who to approach for advice.

## 2.3 The scope of the guidelines

Who are the guidelines for?

These guidelines are intended for the use of managers and those responsible for developing complementary therapy services in organisations which provide supportive and palliative care. Supportive and palliative care is provided in a variety of NHS and non-NHS settings, including hospices, hospitals, primary care, cancer support centres and self-help groups and it is expected that individual service providers will develop local policies and protocols appropriate for their organisation.

What do the guidelines cover?

The purpose of the guidelines is to recommend general principles of best practice, on which services can be developed. These cover the following areas:
- Service development and management
- Practice development

The variety of current operational models, and the different combination of therapies provided in existing services (Kohn 1999, Macmillan 2002) [1] show that services have been developed according to local resources and circumstances, including the vision, enthusiasm and commitment of key individuals. There are vital differences in services, depending on whether provision is in a non-clinical support setting, for example, in the absence of medical or nursing staff, or a clinical hospice or hospital setting. Models, therefore, cannot be imported whole or unchanged and the guidelines provide examples of different configurations of teams (see Appendix A). Various examples are suggested for processes such as referral and assessment, induction, supervision and continuing professional development.

Particular attention is given to the role and recruitment of volunteer therapists as this has been shown to be an area of concern common to most providers currently utilising volunteer therapists within their service.

1 See also The Prince of Wales's Foundation for Integrated Health, 2001 and The Prince of Wales's Foundation for Integrated Health, 2002

Nine therapies have been included: acupuncture, aromatherapy, homeopathy, hypnosis and hypnotherapy, massage, reflexology, reiki, spiritual healing and therapeutic touch. The choice of which therapies to include was based on a number of criteria (see Chapter 12). The information about each therapy includes a brief description, the evidence-base, how they are used in supportive and palliative care, precautions and contraindications and appropriate qualifications. Information is also given about which organisations to contact for advice on therapies less commonly used in palliative and supportive care, such as Bowen technique and shiatsu.

Cancer and three neurological conditions (motor neurone disease, Parkinson's disease and multiple sclerosis) are considered in relation to the use of complementary therapies. Guidance is given about clinical issues that complementary therapists need to be aware of when treating patients with these conditions. Information is also provided on organisations to contact for advice on other progressive, life-limiting or life-threatening conditions, such as heart disease, respiratory conditions and HIV/AIDS.

### What is not covered?
Ernst and Cassileth's (1999) overview of the use of unconventional cancer treatments indicates that such treatments are used, but a distinction is made between alleged cures for cancer itself and preventive and adjunctive measures. In this document, the term complementary therapies refers to those therapies which are used alongside conventional treatment. Alternative treatment options intended to 'cure' cancer are not dealt with in these guidelines.

As indicated, these guidelines are for the use of managers and those responsible for developing complementary therapy services within the NHS and independent sector, including cancer support centres and self-help groups. They are not designed for use as a guide by, or for, patients and the public, nor as a teaching manual for the use of therapies in supportive and palliative care.

## 2.4 Definition of terms

### Complementary therapies
There are several published definitions of the terms complementary medicine and complementary therapy (British Medical Association 1993, Royal College of Nursing 1993, Foundation for Integrated Medicine, 1997). The United States National Institute of Health, Office of Alternative Medicine, coined the term complementary and alternative medicine to encompass both complementary and alternative approaches. This term includes a much broader spectrum of medical and therapeutic approaches to those used in supportive and palliative care.

A distinction is sometimes made between the terms complementary and alternative. Complementary therapies is often used to describe treatments employed alongside, or integrated with, orthodox medical treatment, while alternative therapies indicates those which are used instead, or independently, of orthodox medical treatment (BMA 1993).

In these guidelines, the term complementary therapies refers to those therapies which are used alongside conventional health care.

### Palliative care
The following definition of palliative care, which is based on the World Health Organisation's definition (WHO 1990), and is inclusive of other progressive and life-limiting conditions, has been developed by the National Council for Hospice and Specialist Palliative Care Services (NCHSPCS 2002). This is also the definition proposed in the consultation document of the National Institute for Clinical Excellence (NICE 2002), *Guidance for Cancer Services – Improving Supportive and Palliative Care for Adults with Cancer*.

"Palliative care is the active holistic care of patients with advanced, progressive illness. Management of pain and other symptoms and provision of psychological, social and spiritual support is paramount. The goal of palliative care is achievement of the best quality of life for patients and their families. Many aspects of palliative care are also applicable earlier in the course of the illness in conjunction with other treatments."
(National Council for Hospice and Specialist Palliative Care Services 2002; NICE 2002).

The principles and aims of palliative care are to:
* affirm life and regard dying as a natural process
* provide relief from pain and other symptoms
* integrate the psychological and spiritual aspects of patient care
* offer a support system to help patients live as actively as possible until death
* offer a support system to help the family cope during the patient's illness and in their own bereavement
  *(Aims of Palliative Care*, National Council for Hospice and Specialist Palliative Care Services 2002)

### Supportive care
The concept of supportive care was highlighted in the NHS cancer plan (Department of Health, 2000), when it was also acknowledged that supportive care should be provided throughout patients' and carers' cancer journey. At present the definition and principles of supportive care, as described in *The*

*NHS Cancer Plan*, relate only to cancer services. However, the principles of supportive care are seen to be beneficial for other life-limiting or life-threatening conditions.

Supportive care encompasses nine services, of which complementary therapies is one, that can empower cancer patients and their carers, enable them to develop strategies for living with cancer and support them in the process. The following definition was developed by the National Council for Hospice and Specialist Palliative Care Services (2002) and is also proposed in the National Institute for Clinical Excellence consultation document, *Guidance on Cancer Services – Improving Supportive and Palliative Care for Adults with Cancer* (2002).

"Supportive care is that which helps the patient and their family to cope with cancer and treatment of it – from pre-diagnosis, through the process of diagnosis and treatment, to cure, continuing illness or death and into bereavement. It helps the patient to maximise the benefits of treatment and to live as well as possible with the effects of the disease. It is given equal priority alongside diagnosis and treatment".

The National Council for Hospice and Specialist Palliative Care Services (2002) suggests that there is considerable overlap between supportive and palliative care in terms of need, and that for the usual professional carers of the patient with cancer and their family, this may best be acknowledged by regarding the care they give as supportive/palliative care. The patient's usual professional carers range from the primary care team to professionals within specialist palliative care services, as well as other service providers in the community, such as cancer support centres and support groups.

The range of provider settings and their differing needs and resources have shaped the development of these guidelines as broad principles of best practice on which decisions for developing services can be based. The range of issues considered in the following chapters come under two main headings: service development and management and practice development.

# 3 Development of complementary therapy services

## 3.1 Introduction

This chapter draws on the experience of established services, and considers the issues that are important in the initial stages of service development, as well as in on-going development and management. Depending on the resources of the organisation and the needs of the model adopted, a range of practitioners may provide the hands-on service and corresponding management requirements are suggested. A number of examples are given of the ways in which teams are currently configured.

## 3.2 Initial development: starting up

The initial development of a complementary therapy service is often dependent on the vision of one or more individuals who are prepared to invest time and energy to explore possibilities, and who have the skills to influence development and to take things forward (The Prince of Wales's Foundation for Integrated Health, 2002). What is feasible depends on the resources available, including the skills of existing staff, and the availability of funding, but also on what an organisation considers acceptable funding for starting up a service.

The process of service development can be top down or bottom up or may be an inclusive model where planning and decision-making are shared from the onset. What seems to be important is the creation of an environment that fosters a culture of respect, trust and awareness, which allows the service to evolve and where dialogue and feedback are welcomed (The Prince of Wales's Foundation for Integrated Health, 2002). There are many models of service; but the consensus is that it is advisable to start 'small, safe and simple', and that patient centredness, and the involvement of service users from the beginning, are at the heart of service development. Offering complementary therapies to carers is also seen to be an integral part of caring for patients. Extending the service to staff and volunteers helps to promote the service, as well as provide an element of staff support, which improves working lives.

Consideration needs to be given as to whether patients are required to pay for complementary therapy treatment. Many complementary therapy services in supportive and palliative care are free of

charge; for others a cost is incurred, often based on a sliding scale.

Checklist of issues for consideration in starting a service
- Aims and objectives of the service
- Clarity about approach: top-down, bottom up or inclusive
- Involvement of service users, patients and carers, from the beginning
- Employing a fundraiser
- Funding:
    therapists
    equipment
    therapy space or room
    office space and administration
- Which therapies (see chapters 12-17) and at what point they will be offered
- Accessibility and availability:
    number of sessions
    for patients or patients and carers
    how often
    cultural and language issues
- Consider providing therapies to staff
- Therapists:
    possible configurations of team (see Appendix A)
    recruitment (see chapters 6-7)
    appropriate qualifications (see chapter 5)
    job or role description, person specification
    interview process
- Management should include a designated person to be responsible for overseeing development, and day-to-day management and practicalities (see Table 1 on page 17) including:
    - promoting the availability of the service to - patients, carers and staff
    - familiarising staff with the role of complementary therapies
    - induction, including, where relevant, familiarisation on working within conventional health care setting
    - supervision, appraisal and continuing professional development of therapists (see chapters 4 and 9)
    - policy and protocols (see chapter 4)
    - referral criteria (see chapters 11 – 17)
    - assessment or screening for contraindications (see chapter 11)
    - documentation
    - integration with existing services
    - health and safety measures (see chapter 4)
    - evaluation (see chapter 4)

Initial development: checklist of what works
- involving everyone from the start
- early development of policies, including date for review
- choice and flexibility in service provision
- rigorous recruitment procedures
- a well-developed referral system
- assessment guidelines

- open days for staff in conventional medicine
- providing therapies to staff
- willingness to work within NHS and previous NHS experience
- funding a co-ordinator of complementary therapy services
- supervision
- professionalism
- volunteer training and induction programmes
- sharing good practice
- networking tools such as forums, journals, and meetings

(The Prince of Wales's Foundation for Integrated Health, 2002)

## 3.3 Management and ongoing development

There are many organisational approaches to on-going development, some of which are similar to initial development. Commitment to a patient-centred approach cannot be assumed, and must be underpinned by processes and facilitation which encourage the participation of users at all levels. This challenge requires leadership, a willingness to work collaboratively and the skills to manage change.

Although clinical governance refers primarily to NHS organisations (Department of Health 1999), funders are likely to be looking for similar processes which assure and improve quality in all organisations. Chapter 4 on clinical governance sets out in greater detail the activities that complementary therapy services need to be engaged in.

Two key areas to be considered in on-going development are audit and evaluation, and the introduction of further therapies. Evaluation of a service can result in the following decisions:
a) maintenance of current level of service provision, with simple improvements
b) development of a service that is 'small, safe and simple' into one that is integrated and diverse. Integration can be achieved at different levels, for instance within an organisation and/or in the local area.
c) growth or expansion of the service

When considering the introduction of other therapies, it is important to remember that the lack of evidence does not necessarily constitute evidence of a lack of effectiveness. Where the evidence-base is not strong, often for a variety of reasons, the development of pilot projects, with inbuilt evaluation, would allow the introduction of therapies which could be helpful to patients.

Checklist of ongoing development issues

**Growth or expansion of service**
- Increasing the number of therapies
- Increasing the range of services, for instance groups; classes; teaching therapy skills and self-management skills
- Increasing access, including outreach services to those too ill to leave home; outreach clinics targeting specific groups; bereaved relatives
- Increase in the establishment, such as more therapists
- Maintain or increase funding

**Integration at different levels, within the organisation and in local area**
- Involvement of local community and service users
- Participation at team meetings such as multidisciplinary team, centre team
- Access to patient notes*
- Shared documentation*
- Teaching therapy skills to other members of the clinical team*
- Collaboration and good communication with all involved using letters, telephone calls and meetings
- Recognising the presence of, and relating in ways that overcome, ignorance, prejudice, fear
- Familiarisation with and education in the role of complementary therapies
- Publicity
- Providing a seamless service within local cancer services

**Management and leadership**
- Representation at senior management level*
- Review configuration of team
- Clear lines of responsibility and accountability
- On-going development of therapists, including supervision and appraisal
- Management of change as the service grows, utilising team work and communication
- Management and facilitation of user involvement
- Risk management
- Audit, evaluation and research
- Funding

* in organisations where complementary therapies are offered as part of a multidisciplinary clinical team

## 3.4 Configuration of complementary therapy teams

The configurations of complementary therapy teams are multiple and varied, as are the roles of individuals. Many organisations currently deliver a service by using a combination of employed and volunteer therapists. In a clinical environment, some therapists are also nurses who use complementary therapies alongside their nursing role. Nurses and health care assistants are trained to use therapies in a limited

fashion, for instance simple massage of hands and feet. Other members of the clinical team like doctors, physiotherapists, occupational therapists and social workers may have had additional training in therapies such as acupuncture or Reiki which they incorporate with their primary role.

Services in non-clinical settings are not bound by the same structures as those within the NHS and hospice environments. However, development needs to take into account the absence of on-site support of the clinical team. Cancer patients are also likely to be at an earlier stage of their cancer journey, and may have different needs, such as support during chemotherapy and radiotherapy regimens.

Supportive and palliative care could enhance the rehabilitation of patients with motor neurone disease, Parkinson's disease and multiple sclerosis. Complementary therapies are offered in an integrated way to patients with these conditions, but mainly in hospice settings, and consideration needs to be given as to how they can be provided more widely.

Table 1 indicates the variety of practitioners who may provide complementary therapies within an organisation, and corresponding management requirements.

There are a variety of ways in which services can be developed, depending on resources. What is important is that there are clear lines of accountability and responsibility. Some examples of established teams are shown in Appendix A.

**Table 1** Setting up a service: practitioners and management requirements

| Practitioners | Management requirements |
| --- | --- |
| *Existing staff qualified in complementary therapies to use them with patients on their own caseload or team | Designated individual to take responsibility for<br>• Developing policy, protocols and documentation<br>• Resources and equipment such as essential oils, and acupuncture needles<br>• Supervision |
| *Existing staff who use therapy skills such as simple massage or relaxation with patients on their own caseload or team | Designated individual to take responsibility for<br>• Recruitment<br>• Training and supervising staff<br>• Developing policy and protocols<br>• Equipment such as essential oils |
| Paid full-time, part-time, sessional or self-employed or volunteer therapists | Designated individual to take responsibility for<br>• Recruitment including job or role description<br>• Contract or written agreement<br>• Office and equipment<br>• Therapy room(s)<br>• Induction, supervision and training appropriate to the experience of the therapist<br>• Developing policy, protocols and documentation<br>• Equipment such as oils, sheets and towels, couch or acupuncture needles<br>• Coordinating practical issues such as referrals, working days and therapy space<br>• Supervision and appraisal |
| Volunteer therapy assistants | Designated individual to take responsibility for<br>• Recruitment including role description<br>• Contract or written agreement<br>• Induction, training and supervision<br>• Developing policy, protocols and documentation<br>• Equipment such as essential oils<br>• Co-ordinating practical issues, for example referrals, working days and therapy space<br>• Supervision and appraisal |
| Complementary therapies coordinator, who is also a provider | Designated individual to take management responsibility for:<br>• Recruiting the coordinator<br>• Contract of employment<br>• Office and equipment<br>• Identifying a therapy room or space<br>• Induction and supervision<br>• Priorities for service development |

*Applies to clinical settings only; existing staff refers to members of the clinical team with conventional healthcare roles

# 4 Clinical governance

## 4.1 Introduction

Clinical governance is the framework through which NHS organisations are accountable for continuously improving the quality of their services and safeguarding high standards of care, by creating an environment where excellence will flourish (Department of Health 1998). Although this framework applies to NHS organisations, it is equally important for services in the voluntary sector to demonstrate to funders and others their determination to safeguard quality of care. This chapter considers the importance of clinical governance for complementary therapy services, within and outside of the NHS. The different aspects of clinical governance addressed include the development of policies, supervision, appraisal, continuing professional development, audit evaluation and research, and risk management.

The white paper, *The new NHS: Modern, Dependable* (DoH 1997) and the consultation document *A First Class Service: quality in the new NHS* (DoH 1998) set out the government's strategy for ensuring that quality of care becomes the driving force for the development of health services in England. Central to this is clinical governance. Voluntary sector hospices are already very familiar with the concept of quality improvement, and 48% have started to implement clinical governance (NCHSPCS 2002a). The National Council for Hospice and Specialist Palliative Care Services has provided guidance on how the principles of clinical governance may be applied to voluntary sector hospices (NCHSPCS 2000), and how some hospices have interpreted clinical governance according to their own needs (NCHSPCS 2002a).

The principles of quality improvement apply equally to complementary therapy services, and many services may already be pursuing quality improvement activities. The challenge posed by the duty of quality of care, in complementary therapies, is to review and transform the delivery of services so that:
- patients are included in planning and evaluation
- there is written information for patients about the different therapies provided, how they may help, how to access the service and complaints procedures
- decisions on choice of therapy and/or the aims of treatment are based on the best available evidence
- consistently better outcomes are produced for patients
- there is a reduction in variations of access, so that issues such as geographical location, needs of housebound patients and promoting the service with minority groups are considered
- there is a collaborative style of leadership, systems awareness, teamwork and effective communication
- there are clear procedures to enable staff to report any concerns about colleagues' professional conduct or performance

The main components of clinical governance, as applied in the NHS, are set out in Appendix B. The activities within the framework of clinical governance recommended for complementary therapy services are described in the following sections.

## 4.2 Policies, procedures and standards

These national guidelines have also been developed to form a reference point for the development of local policies, procedures and standards. Many organisations have already developed policies and procedures. It may be useful for those developing policies to look at the policies and procedures of other organisations, in order to choose the elements which most nearly meet local needs.

Policies are agreed rules that the organisation makes to ensure safe and consistent practice, and to reduce risk. Policies clearly outline what staff need to do, as well as limits, so that staff understand what is expected of them. When drawing up policies the place of professional judgement should be considered. (See also Chapter 8 on professional and ethical issues)

Procedures describe how to do something, outlining in considerable detail the elements of good practice that should be followed to achieve a quality result.

Standards are statements which distil elements of good practice, a measure against which quality can be judged, so as to ensure that procedures have been followed. Standards often extract elements of good practice from procedures.

## 4.3 Supervision

This is addressed separately in Chapter 9 on supervision.

## 4.4 Individual performance review or appraisal

Individual performance review or appraisal is a strategy that encourages professional and personal development and contributes to quality,

improvement of services and the development of an organisation. Many organisations have established procedures for this process. When fully understood and implemented, it is a two-way process, which can both motivate and support staff. It is recommended that all organisations which employ therapists develop a system for appraising or reviewing performance.

## 4.5 Education and training

Continuing professional development (CPD) is a requirement for on-going registration of many complementary therapy professions, and has also been identified as a quality improvement activity within clinical governance.

Education and training needs vary, depending on existing skills and experience. The needs of complementary therapy staff for specialist training to work in palliative care should be assessed and planned for. Chapter 10 on clinical issues is a resource that can be used when considering the CPD needs of therapists working in supportive and palliative care. Training in assessment, communication and counselling skills can also improve quality of care. (See Chapter 9 on supervision, and Chapter 11 on referral and assessment).

Several organisations offer comprehensive programmes of training for complementary therapists working in palliative care, parts of which may be accessible in independent modules. Courses are available in different parts of England, including Bristol, East Sussex, London, Manchester, and Rochdale.

## 4.6 Audit and evaluation

Clinical governance encourages an evaluation culture, which measures effectiveness in the form of patient outcomes. Audit of different aspects of service delivery, for example waiting times, uptake of service, responsiveness of service, missed appointments, cost and adverse events, can inform planning and delivery. However, the primary role of audit and evaluation of complementary therapy services in supportive and palliative care is to seek the views of patients, as well as measuring outcomes, on a regular and systematic basis.

The difficulty of identifying a single tool which captures the whole picture of how patients may be benefitting from complementary therapies is recognised and is an area for future research. The following section on research suggests a range of methodologies and other resources can be found in Appendix C.

## 4.7 Research and development

Clinical governance encourages participation in well-designed, relevant research and development activities. Research is essential for the improvement and broadening of services and skills in all branches of the health professions and palliative care (Franks & Ahmedzai 1995). However, the difficulties of conducting research in complementary therapies and supportive and palliative care are acknowledged and include funding, ethical issues, high attrition rates and lack of research experience amongst complementary therapy practitioners. (House of Lords 2000; Westcombe et al in press)

The diversity of patients' symptoms and experience and the complex nature of complementary therapy interventions provide a challenge. A single methodological approach is unlikely to provide evidence of the spectrum of potential benefits for patients. A multifaceted approach is recommended, which is inclusive of:
- Objective measures in relation to, for example, sleep, nausea and vomiting, need for medication, use of other services, cost-effectiveness
- Subjective measures to assess pain, quality of life, well-being, anxiety, depression
- Exploration of the patient's experience and concerns

If research, rather than evaluation of services, is undertaken it is important to take into account the difficulties that may arise. These include attempting to match sample populations, patients being at different stages of illness and patients having different types of cancer. It is also important to be aware of the implications of conclusions that may be drawn. In the absence of in-house expertise in research, it may be helpful to work with the local university health research department.

Standardised and validated questionnaires and other audit tools which are used in cancer and palliative care include:
- Hospital Anxiety and Depression Scale (Zigmond and Snaith 1983)
- Rotterdam Symptom Checklist (De Haes et al 1990)
- State-Trait Anxiety Inventory (Spielberger et al 1983)
- Quality of life and symptom distress scale (Holmes and Dickerson 1987)
- Measure Your Medical Outcome Profile (Paterson 1996; Paterson & Britten 2000)
- Measure Your Concerns and Well-Being (Paterson et al 2002)

A number of databases can be used to search for published research on complementary therapies. The list compiled by Richardson (2001) can be seen in Appendix D.

## 4.8 Health and Safety

Organisational policies aimed at assessing and managing risks should be understood by all complementary therapists. In complementary therapy services, issues for consideration include the following:

- Training in safe handling and moving
- Risk assessment
- Reporting of critical incidents which ensures that adverse events are identified, investigated, and lessons are learned and applied
- Disposal of equipment, such as acupuncture needles, and essential oil containers
- Storage of essential oils, acupuncture equipment and homeopathic remedies
- Spillage of essential oils

# 5 Regulation and training of complementary therapists

## 5.1 Introduction

The training and qualification of therapists is a key issue for managers. The Prince of Wales's Foundation for Integrated Health is supporting a number of therapies in their development of a more robust system of regulation and accreditation of training for their professions. This chapter outlines the current position on regulation and training, and gives information which may be useful for the appointment of therapists.

## 5.2 Regulation: the current position

With the exception of osteopaths and chiropractors, who are regulated by law, (statute) most complementary therapy practice is either voluntarily self-regulated or is unregulated. In response to the House of Lords Report (2000), the government strongly encouraged the representative bodies within each therapy to unite to form a single body for regulating their profession (Department of Health 2001). This approach is considered to be in the best interests of patients and the wider public, as well as potentially enhancing the status of individual professions. The acupuncture and herbal medicine professions have formed working groups to develop proposals for statutory regulation. Some professions have well-developed voluntary self-regulatory structures and others are working towards that position.

Most of the therapies included in these guidelines are working to achieve statutory or voluntary self-regulation and have formed working groups to make proposals for the development of single regulatory bodies for their profession. The working groups are currently at different stages of development. However, they are likely to play an increasingly important role in developing self-regulation, including overseeing standards of education and training.

All practitioners of complementary healthcare are advised to register with an organisation that ensures its members are properly qualified, insured to practise, and undertake continuing professional development. Membership of a professional organisation represented on the working group for developing a single regulatory body for the profession is likely to assume increasing importance.

A professional organisation should have:
- High quality, clear information on its registrants and what they offer
- Membership requirements which include competence to practise and insurance
- Requirements for renewal of membership which include continuing professional development
- A code of conduct and practice
- Complaints and disciplinary procedures
- A system for involving members in decision-making
- Published annual accounts

### Conventional healthcare professionals

Statutorily regulated health professionals such as doctors, nurses and physiotherapists who wish to practise complementary therapies are bound by the code of conduct of their profession. However, they are advised to consult their regulatory body (eg Nursing and Midwifery Council), their professional body (eg Royal College of Nursing) and employer for guidance before incorporating complementary therapies into their clinical practice. Organisations which offer healthcare within the NHS and the independent sector are advised to develop local policies and protocols for the use of complementary therapies.

The government's response to the House of Lords Select Committee report on complementary and alternative medicine recommended that each statutory regulatory body in the conventional healthcare professions, whose members make significant use of complementary therapies, should develop clear guidelines for members on both the competences and training required for the safe and effective practice of the leading complementary therapies. (Department of Health 2001)

The Chartered Society of Physiotherapists (CSP) have published an information paper on physiotherapy and complementary medicine (CSP 2002). Massage, as a manual therapy, remains a core skill of many chartered physiotherapists. Individual physiotherapists are increasingly integrating a range of complementary therapy approaches into their own scope of practice, and there are a number of clinical complementary therapy interest groups recognised by the CSP. (www.csp.org.uk)

The Royal College of Nursing and the Nursing and Midwifery Council have issued guidelines on practice for nurses thinking about some of the issues around complementary therapies (for example see www.rcn.org.uk). Advice is given about
- Indemnity insurance for practitioners using complementary therapies
- Product liability cover
- Self-employed practitioners using complementary

therapies
- Nurses who work as homeopaths
- Choosing a complementary therapy course
- Advertising
- Homeopathic substances and herbal preparations

## 5.3 Training, qualifications and national occupational standards

Courses in osteopathy and chiropractic, which are statutorily regulated therapies, are standardised and accredited by the regulatory bodies for each therapy. Many of the other complementary professions are working towards common standards of education and training and the accreditation of professional courses. The government has recommended that any accreditation board is completely independent of the institutions being accredited. (Departmen of Health 2001).

For conventional healthcare practitioners, the government supports the recommendation (House of Lords 2000) that the training of these professionals should be to standards agreed with the appropriate complementary therapy regulatory body (Department of Health 2001). This may include the development of standards which reflect both training and practice at different levels.

Complementary therapy qualifications
A qualification may be
- a diploma or other qualification awarded by a private college or training institute
- a nationally recognised qualification, such as a diploma, from an awarding body that is regulated by one of the four UK statutory regulating authorities. These are:
  - for England, the Qualifications and Curriculum Authority (QCA)
  - for Wales, the Qualifications, Curriculum and Assessment Authority (ACCAC), except for national vocational qualifications, which are regulated by the QCA
  - for Scotland, the Scottish Qualifications Authority (SQA)
  - for Northern Ireland, the Council for the Curriculum, Examinations and Assessments (CCEA), except for post-19 external qualifications which are regulated by the QCA.
- a degree, or sometimes a higher certificate or diploma, from a university

For details of the external awarding bodies for complementary therapy qualifications currently regulated by the QCA please see the QCA website www.qca.org.uk

National occupational standards are statements of competence, and are written to measure performance outcomes. Competence may be described as the ability to apply knowledge, understanding and skills in performing to the standards required in employment. National occupational standards describe good practice, are used by providers of education and training to define learning outcomes, and form a basis for qualifications.

National occupational standards are published by the Qualifications and Curriculum Authority. At the time of publication of these guidelines, standards have been published for aromatherapy, homeopathy, hypnotherapy and reflexology and are being developed for other therapies. For information on the progress of national occupational standards for other therapies, contact Skills for Health, the national training organisation for health (www.skillsforhealth.co.uk), which is contracted by the Qualifications and Curriculum Authority to develop and set standards.

## 5.4 Choosing a therapist: qualifications and regulation

Membership of a professional organisation represented on the working group developing a single regulatory body for individual therapies is likely to assume increasing importance. Appendix E provides the following information about the therapies included in these guidelines:
- The working groups for the development of single regulatory bodies for each therapy, with lists of member organisations (as at May 2003).
- The availability of national occupational standards for each therapy.

However, if therapists do not belong to one of these organisations the interview process will assume particular importance for verification of competence. This may include, for example, using competency-based questions or scenarios. Please see Chapter 6.4 on interview and assessment.

It is in the interests of services and therapists that therapists are registered with organisations that are represented on developing working groups if there is one for that therapy.

# 6 Recruitment and Selection

## 6.1 Introduction

The purpose of this chapter is to provide information that will be useful when employing complementary therapists. Key points to be considered include the candidate's prior experience in supportive and palliative care, their experience of using the therapy, assessment of competence and other skills. Orientation and induction complete the recruitment process. The qualification and regulation of therapists is an area of particular concern to employers and Chapter 5 is devoted to this subject. This chapter should be considered in conjunction with Chapter 7 on volunteer therapists.

## 6.2 Regulation and training

When considering the qualifications of therapists reference should be made to Chapter 5 for the current position on regulation and training.

## 6.3 Prior experience

It is reasonable to expect complementary therapy coordinators or team leaders and other therapists who are paid, to have had education, training or experience of working in supportive and palliative care, and of using complementary therapies with people who are ill. Relevant experience would be desirable for volunteer therapists but training and supervision can be provided, if there is a complementary therapy coordinator or team leader. (See Chapter 7 on volunteers)

## 6.4 Interview and assessment

The interview process is crucial in the recruitment and selection of therapists, particularly since there are at present variable standards of training in many therapies. Patients emphasise the need for a therapist to be a 'people person' and have excellent interpersonal and communication skills, as well as being appropriately qualified. (The Prince of Wales's Foundation for Integrated Health 2002) It is advisable to include a service user on the interview panel, as well as an experienced practitioner in the therapy for which the candidate is being interviewed. Some organisations incorporate in the interview an assessment of the skills and strengths of the therapist. For example, the applicant may be required to give a short treatment to a member of the panel who takes the role of the patient.

Recruitment and selection: best practice key points

a) Organisations should have a recruitment and selection policy that includes equal opportunities and which is communicated to all staff

b) Systems must be fair, consistent and valid

c) Recruitment and selection must take into account the needs of the individual as well as the needs of the organisation

d) All applications should be acknowledged where possible and treated confidentially

e) Recruitment advertisements should:
* state briefly the requirements of the job and the necessary and desirable criteria for job applicants
* state the activities and working practices of the organisation
* state the job location, and application procedure
* state the reward package, and job tenure
* not make misleading claims or present misleading information
* never contain age barriers or age-related criteria

f) Job profiles and person specifications should:
* outline roles and responsibilities
* state the necessary and desirable criteria for selection
* be based on appropriate qualifications and competencies, for example skills, aptitude, knowledge and experience
* specify the personal qualities relevant to the job, such as the ability to work as part of a team (See Appendix F for an example of a job description for a complementary therapy co-ordinator)

g) References
* The recruitment policy should state clearly how references will be used, at what stage of the recruitment process, and what kind of referees will be necessary. These rules should be applied consistently
* Recruiters should always use references to check factual information, such as qualifications
* Former employers should not be asked to supply a subjective opinion as to an applicant's likely future performance

h) Occupational health clearance and medical examinations
* It is reasonable to require the completion of a health questionnaire where good health is relevant to the job
* Public service organisations are obliged to obtain occupational health clearance for a prospective employee

i) Criminal Records Bureau
* Clearance for new staff working with children and vulnerable adults must be obtained from 1 April

2002 and for existing staff by April 2004 (Department of Health 2000).

j) Interviews should:
* always be conducted or supervised by trained individuals
* be structured to follow a previously agreed set of questions mirroring the personal specifications or job profile
* allow candidates the opportunity to ask questions

It is desirable to include on the interview panel a service user and an experienced practitioner in the therapy for which the candidate is being interviewed. (Chartered Institute of Personnel Development 2002)

## 6.5 Salary

The payment of therapists varies widely. The salary of team leaders or coordinators can vary from about £17,000 – £30,000 per annum. Posts which have been incorporated in the nursing budget are paid according to the nursing scale and can range from grade E – grade H. Self-employed therapists are paid per session and this can vary from £10-£30 per hour.

Leadership roles include team leader, lecturer-practitioner, lecturer and consultant. It is recommended that posts should be graded according to the role expected of the post-holder. The job descriptions of therapists should be comparable to those of other members of the clinical team (if any) in terms of skills and responsibilities required and posts should be graded accordingly.

## 6.6 Contract

It is a legal requirement for employers to provide employees with a contract stating the terms and conditions of employment. Self-employed therapists should also have a contract which states terms and conditions, including agreements regarding payment when appointments are cancelled. It may be important to include ethical issues such as confidentiality, not making claims about outcomes and not criticising or judging other health professionals. (See Chapter 8 on professional and ethical issues)

## 6.7 Orientation and induction

Therapists should receive the same orientation as that provided for other members of the clinical team. The induction needs of therapists differ and should be agreed and planned with the individual. Information on precautions to be taken when providing treatment in supportive and palliative care can be found in Chapters 12-17 on the therapies, but this should not be used in place of additional specialist training. Therapists should be introduced to all the policies and procedures of the organisation, including personnel and health and safety policies.

# 7 Volunteer Therapists

## 7.1 Introduction

There are a number of organisations in supportive and palliative care which depend on volunteer therapists. The use, recruitment and management of volunteer therapists are issues which generate much debate (The Prince of Wales's Foundation for Integrated Health 2002). One of the key points in working with volunteers is the principle of reciprocity, which can often be overlooked in a busy workplace. This chapter considers the issues involved in managing volunteer therapists, such as recruitment terminology, line management, supervision and support, and gives information on best practice.

On the one hand best practice demands the development of a culture that values the contribution of volunteers. On the other hand, the management of volunteer therapists is time consuming and has to be balanced against the benefits. It is said of the voluntary sector that "individuals and teams of paid staff and volunteers are striving to accomplish an enormous amount with resources that are never sufficient" (Voluntary Sector National Training Organisation 2002). This is true for all organisations delivering health care. Time and expertise, therefore, are at a premium and "volunteers are a source of risk or liability as well as a benefit". (Association of Chief Executives of Voluntary Organisations 1998)

A well-managed volunteer service can deliver benefit to the organisation and also to the volunteer in terms of personal satisfaction. The home office and the National Council for Voluntary Organisations have developed a code of good practice for volunteering in general. (NCVO 2001) Some of the basic points are summarised in Appendix G. Supported by the Department of Education and Skills, the voluntary sector national training organisation is taking the NCVO *Volunteering: Code of Good Practice* forward in a project to develop national occupational standards for managing volunteers. (Voluntary Sector National Training Organisation 2002) The project is due for completion by September 2003, and information can be obtained from the Voluntary Sector National Training Organisation website www.voluntarysectorskills.org.uk

One of the principles of volunteering is reciprocity: volunteers offer their contribution unwaged, but should benefit in return. Benefits to volunteers include the establishment of a reciprocal relationship in which the volunteer gains a sense of worthwhile achievement, experience and contacts; is taught the skills involved in the execution of their role, and is

included in the life of the organisation. It should be recognised that volunteer complementary therapists are highly qualified individuals who are either financially in a position to give some of their time freely and are motivated to do so, and/or want to gain experience while building up a private practice or waiting for paid employment opportunities.

The following key areas, which need to be considered in managing complementary therapy volunteers, are addressed in this section:
- Recruitment and selection
- Orientation and induction
- Line management
- Supervision and support
- Professional and ethical issues
- Continuing relationships with patients and carers
- Application of personnel policies
- Health and safety

## 7.2 Recruitment and selection

### Qualifications
The qualifications of volunteer therapists should be no less than those required of paid therapists (see Chapter 5 on regulation and training).

### Role description and agreement
In order to be clear about the expectations of a volunteer therapist and encourage belonging within the organisation, it is suggested that volunteers should receive a role description as part of the recruitment process. An example of a role description is found in Appendix H. However, there has been increasing litigation in relation to volunteering, following recent developments in employment law. Role descriptions should be free of any terms which can be construed as employment terminology, such as job description, hours of work, probation, appraisal and obligations. It is also advisable to be clear that there is no intention to create a legally binding relationship. For advice, organisations should contact their legal advisers, the Citizens Advice Bureau, the National Council for Voluntary Organisations, or the Employment Law Help Line of Help the Hospices.

### Process
The principles of best practice which apply to the employment of paid therapists should be adhered to in the recruitment of volunteers (see Chapter 6 on recruitment). For example, there should be a process through which qualifications, insurance and references are checked and an interview which provides the opportunity for judging the suitability of therapists for working in supportive and palliative care, and which could include an assessment of skills. Public service organisations are obliged to obtain occupational health clearance for individuals. Clearance for working with children and vulnerable

adults, as an employee or volunteer of any organisation, must be obtained for new staff (paid or volunteer) from 1 April 2002 and for existing staff by April 2004 (Department of Health 2000).

### Agreements

Volunteering agreements, including details of the placement, should be confirmed in writing (Voluntary Sector National Training Organisation 2002). However, as for the role description, it is important to avoid any terms which could be construed as employment terminology.

## 7.3 Orientation and induction

A volunteer therapist should receive a general orientation to the organisation, and the complementary therapy service. Specific induction needs should be identified with the individual, and planned for. Additional training may be required, for instance in supportive and palliative care, the use of the specific therapy in supportive and palliative care or working in a conventional health care setting, a non-clinical environment or in a patient's home. Organisations with volunteer therapists and/or whose in-house expertise does not extend to teaching the use of complementary therapies in palliative care should consider paying for short courses or study days provided by other organisations.

## 7.4 Line management

Volunteer therapists should be introduced to the structure of the organisation so that they can see where they fit in. Line management responsibilities should be clarified. Regular planned reviews can be used to identify supervision and support needs, assess satisfaction levels, reassess the availability of the volunteer versus the needs of the organisation to provide a service and clarify the time commitment involved in managing volunteers.

## 7.5 Supervision and support

The expectation that volunteer therapists should participate in supervision can be difficult to fulfil. Volunteer therapists have been known to be motivated to give their time freely to patients and carers, but less keen to participate in supervision for themselves. (The Prince of Wales's Foundation for Integrated Health 2002) Nevertheless, supervision could be provided in-house or the individual could be responsible for their own therapy specific supervision and reflective practice away from the

organisation (see Chapter 9 on supervision). Management supervision should be via the therapist's line manager within the organisation.

Support can be provided in a variety of other ways, for example informally, through network groups or peer support, and through opportunities to receive and exchange therapies. Supporting the development of volunteers' knowledge, skills and competence can be done through participation in in-house study days, discussion groups, involvement in planning and evaluation, and through innovative projects.

## 7.6 Code of practice

Volunteer therapists are bound by the code of practice of the professional organisation of which they are members. They should be accountable for their practice and behaviour in the same way that paid therapists are. Details are given in the separate section on professional and ethical issues in Chapter 8. In addition, organisations should have, or develop, their own policies on issues such as confidentiality, consent, and the receipt of gifts.

## 7.7 Continuing relationships with patients and carers

A contentious issue seems to be the continuation of a professional relationship between the volunteer therapist and the patient or carer, once the person has completed their treatment in the organisation (The Prince of Wales's Foundation for Integrated Health 2002). Patients value continuity once they have established a relationship with a therapist, and find the continuation of the professional relationship a support for their illness journey.

Concerns regarding the continuation of treatment in a private capacity with the therapist include lack of supervision of the therapist in relation to the patient's changing clinical condition, issues of accountability, and legal and ethical issues where the patient sees the continuation of treatment as a continuation of the service provided by the organisation. For example, a patient could subsequently involve the organisation in a complaint about the treatment or therapist.

It is recommended that organisations consider this issue and are clear about where they stand, and for that position to be made clear to potential therapists. However, it is the patient's right to negotiate where and from whom they receive private treatment. A way forward may be that when such a situation

occurs, the patient should be clear that he/she is entering into a private contract with the therapist, and that this is unconnected with the organisation.

It is also recommended that organisations consider compiling a list of therapists in the local area with experience of treating people with cancer and/or chronic illness. This list could be made available for patients, although it would be important to emphasise that the list should not be interpreted as a recommendation of therapists by the organisation.

## 7.8 Personnel policies

Personnel policies which apply specifically to volunteers, and other general policies that also apply to volunteers, should be easily accessible to the volunteer. These policies should include:
- Equal opportunities, diversity, and anti-discriminatory statements
- Complaints policy
- Management of capability, skills and development
- Staff support policies
- Disciplinary and grievance policy
- Bullying and harassment policy

Policies should provide volunteers with information about the organisation's expectations and the requirements of their role. Details of support and protection for the volunteer should be included.

## 7.9 Health and safety

Volunteer therapists should be familiarised with the health and safety policies of the organisation, and should be included in annual safe handling and moving training and fire training.

# 8 Professional and Ethical Issues

## 8.1 Introduction

Although professional organisations that register complementary therapists should have codes of practice and ethics, the multitude of organisations that currently exist for many therapies results in as many different codes and varying standards. This chapter has adapted standards for professional accountability, consent and confidentiality from the medical, nursing and midwifery professions. It is recommended that complementary therapy professionals working in supportive and palliative care and who are not also a member of a statutorily regulated profession, should follow these standards, in addition to those set by their own professional organisation.

Although these guidelines have drawn on the documents, *Code of Professional Conduct* (Nursing and Midwifery Council 2002a), *Standards of Practice* (General Medical Council 1998), *Duties of a Doctor* (General Medical Council 1998) and other documents (Nursing and Midwifery Council 2002 b-e), it is emphasised that the adaptation of these medical and nursing standards does not in any way imply that either the General Medical Council or Nursing and Midwifery Council has responsibility for complementary practitioners. The regulation of doctors, nurses, midwives and health visitors is separate from the ethical standards recommended in these guidelines for complementary therapists. Moreover, the recommendation of the following ethical standards does not imply a similar level of expertise, training or regulation of non-statutorily regulated complementary therapists.

## 8.2 Professional accountability

Ethical guidance aims to promote optimal standards of care (Stone 2002). As a general rule, the complementary therapist shall act, at all times, in such a manner as to:
* safeguard and promote the interests and well-being of clients
* justify the trust and confidence of clients
* uphold and enhance the good standing and reputation of their complementary therapy profession
* uphold and enhance the good standing of the organisation in which they are providing a service

Complementary therapists are personally accountable for their practice, and in the exercise of that professional accountability, must :

* ensure that no action or omission on their part is detrimental to the interests, condition or safety of clients
* maintain and improve their professional knowledge and competence
* recognise the limits of their professional competence
* make no claims for their treatment which are not wholly true and justifiable
* communicate and provide information in a way that clients can understand
* work in partnership with clients, foster their independence, and respect the treatment choices they make
* respond to patients' need for care, irrespective of gender, age, race, disability, sexuality, culture or religious beliefs
* maintain professional boundaries and avoid any abuse of their privileged relationship with clients and of the privileged access allowed to the client's person, property or residence.
* protect all confidential information concerning clients obtained in the course of professional practice and make disclosures only with consent, or within the policy of confidentiality as practised within the organisation, except where they can justify disclosure in the wider public interest
* refuse any gift, favour or hospitality from clients currently in their care which might be interpreted as seeking to exert influence to obtain preferential consideration
* work in a collaborative and co-operative manner with the multidisciplinary team and others involved in providing care
* recognise and respect the role and contribution of colleagues, within conventional medicine and other complementary therapy practitioners; for example, when interacting with a client do not criticise or question any other colleague's approach
* report to an appropriate person or authority any circumstances which could jeopardise or compromise safety or standards of practice, including the fitness of themselves or a colleague to practice, while having regard to the physical, psychological and social effects on clients
* follow the employing organisation's policies and protocols

## 8.3 Consent

There are three over-riding professional responsibilities with regard to obtaining consent. The practitioner must:
* act in the best interests of the client
* ensure that the process of establishing consent is transparent and demonstrates a clear level of professional accountability
* record all discussions and decisions accurately

Valid consent consists of three elements:
- if the patient is unable to give consent themselves, it is given by a competent person, who may be a person lawfully appointed on behalf of the patient
- it is informed
- it is given voluntarily

Effective communication is the key to enabling clients to make informed decisions, and includes finding out about the individual's needs and priorities. Sufficient information should be provided, in a way that the client can understand, and this includes an explanation of any risks involved. Sufficient time needs to be set aside for this, so that the individual has the time to consider and ask questions before making a decision.

A client who is legally competent may give consent in writing, verbally or by co-operation. Some organisations prefer to have written consent to complementary therapy treatment. Other organisations consider verbal consent, or consent by implication (by cooperating) to be sufficient. The complementary therapist should follow the policy of the organisation with regard to written or verbal consent. In the case of verbal consent therapists should record their discussion with the client at the time of the assessment.

The scope of consent should be clear. For example, a client who consents to having reflexology, has not also consented to receiving acupuncture. This should also be made clear to the patient.

The policy of the organisation should be followed in cases where the patient is semi-conscious or unconscious and unable to give consent. If a client declines treatment at any particular time, this should be respected and recorded.

When complementary therapies are provided in an organisation where there is a medical team, for instance within the NHS or a hospice in-patient unit, the patient's doctor has the overall legal responsibility for the patient's care. A system for obtaining consent from the patient's doctor for the use of the different complementary therapies should be agreed.

## 8.4 Confidentiality

The therapist should recognise and respect a client's right to expect that information given in confidence will be used only for the purpose for which it was given, and will not be released to others without their permission.

The therapist is responsible for any decision to release confidential information. If it is appropriate to share information gained in the course of giving treatment with other health and social work colleagues, the therapist must ensure that as far as is reasonable, the information will be kept in strict professional confidence and used only for the purpose for which it was given.

As it is impractical to obtain consent every time information needs to be shared with others, the therapist should ensure that the client understands from the start that some information may be made available to other members of the team involved in the delivery of care. In some organisations this is known as team confidentiality. The therapist should follow the organisation's policy on confidentiality. Disclosure of information, without consent and outside of the team, may be made only where it can be justified in the public interest, usually where disclosure is essential to protect the client or someone else from the risk of significant harm, or when the therapist is required by law or by order of a court. Clients should be made aware of this.

With regard to disclosure of information where there is an issue of child protection, the therapist should act at all times in accordance with national and local policies.

# 9 Supervision

## 9.1 Introduction

Supervision is understood to be central to the process of learning before expansion of the scope of practice and a means of encouraging assessment, analytical and reflective skills. (Department of Health 1993) There are different interpretations of the terms supervision and clinical supervision. This chapter describes supervision which is specific to the practice of the particular therapy and that which facilitates reflection on practice. Suggestions are made about the different ways in which supervision can be organised, but managers and therapists need to be clear about how the cost of supervision will be met.

As a formal process of professional support and learning, supervision:
- enables individual practitioners to develop knowledge and skills to help them meet new challenges, find ways of meeting needs and remain receptive to change through the development of practice
- provides support for those working in stressful and distressing situations
- maintains high standards of safe and effective care
  (Department of Health 1993; NHS Executive 1994)

The benefits of supervision have been reported in different studies (Bowles & Young 1999; Cullverwell & Green 1998), but the evidence to support supervision for complementary therapies is currently largely anecdotal or derived from a small number of studies. (Mackereth 2001)

Whilst supervision is also considered to be an effective risk management tool (Tingle 1995), for it to be welcomed and effective it must also be viewed as useful, safe and appropriate to the supervisee's practice. (Mackereth1997) Within complementary therapies, depending on the therapy practised and the structure of provision of supervision within an organisation, supervision can be further sub-divided into the provision of therapy specific supervision and reflective practice, although in some situations this distinction is not made.

## 9.2 Therapy specific supervision

Therapy specific supervision is supervision in the use of a particular therapy in the context of supportive and palliative care. This can also be understood as an exchange between practising professionals to enable the development of professional skills. (Faugier and Butterworth 1994) The depth of supervision depends on the therapist's experience of practising the therapy, of working with patients, and of using the therapy within supportive and palliative care. It is suggested that organisations should assess the therapist's experience and expertise in the interviewing process, agree the level of supervision required and agree who will provide this. If the organisation is unable to provide therapy specific supervision, for instance, for an acupuncturist, it may be that the therapist will need to find an external supervisor. Some employers specify that self employed therapists are responsible for their own therapy specific supervision.

## 9.3 Supervision as reflection on practice

### Purpose
The purpose of providing time, space and a supportive relationship that enables practitioners to reflect on their own practice is two-fold. Firstly, the motives for working in the helping or caring professions are not clear and simple, and the role of helper carries with it certain expectations. (Hawkins and Shohet 1989) Supervision can improve patient care by distinguishing personal from professional issues, thus enabling the focus to remain on the patient, while supporting practitioners in work that can be challenging and emotionally demanding. Other benefits include an increase in confidence, and the avoidance of burnout. (Hallberg et al 1994) Developing clear supervision contracts, and ensuring that supervisors also receive supervision for their role, can contribute to clarifying the boundaries within supervision. (Mackereth 2001)

Secondly, the provision of supervision acknowledges and celebrates the potency in therapeutic work. (Mackereth 1997) Emotional and physical responses to complementary therapy treatments can happen. The practitioner's skills and support, and issues of boundaries to practice need to be considered in order to effectively manage any emotional and physical responses. (Mackereth 1999) Complementary therapists usually see patients on a one to one basis, and additional training in communication skills may increase their confidence when relating to patients in challenging situations. Studies have shown that communication skills can be taught, (cited in Heaven & Maguire 1997) and there is growing evidence to support effective models for training in communication skills. (National Institute for Clinical Excellence 2002)

### Training in communication skills
Training programmes in communication skills that lead to positive outcomes should:
- include cognitive, behavioural and emotional aspects of communication and focus on the

acquisition of specific skills and/or strategies for dealing with specific situations
- use a combination of didactic and experiential methods, including role play, group work and discussion
- be learner centred
- provide a safe environment for the development of skills, reflection and self-awareness
- have defined and measurable core competencies
- be led by professionals who are trained and understand issues relevant to the clinical context
- provide constructive feedback
  (National Institute for Clinical Excellence 2002)

The following are examples of communication skills training currently available:
- Cancer Research UK, Psychological Medicine Group, Stanley House, Christie Hospital NHS Trust, Wilmslow Road, Manchester M20 4BX. Tel: 0161 446 3679. Facilitated by Professor Peter Maguire and team
- Help the Hospices, Hospice House, 34-44 Britannia Street, London WC1X 9JG. Tel: 020 7520 8200. Facilitated by Dr. Susie Wilkinson and Anita Roberts
- St. Ann's Hospice, Institute for Learning and Development, St. Ann's Road North, Heald Green, Cheadle, Cheshire SK8 3SZ. Tel: 0161 437 8136. Contact Christine Lawther, Head of the Institute for Learning and Development

### The culture of supervision
Apart from the social work and counselling professions, the culture of supervision within the helping professions is not strong. Indeed, the need for supervision has often been regarded negatively, as an acknowledgement of weakness. However, one of the implications of the introduction of clinical governance is the need to create an environment for life-long learning, in which excellence will flourish. Within this culture, the understanding of the value of supervision is growing, although it is still early days. The issues that need to be considered are:
- a general lack of experience of the supervision process in the helping professions, both of supervisees and supervisors
- the provision of supervision to therapists working in diverse settings and circumstances, such as self-employed, sessional, part-time, volunteers, hospitals, cancer support groups, self-help groups
- a general reluctance by professionals to engage in the supervision process for a variety of reasons, some of which are personal, financial or professional, not least a lack of understanding of the value of supervision
- management support for developing supervision.

### The organisation of supervision
As there is no statutory requirement for supervision, the challenge to introducing this supportive and professional development strategy demands flexible

models that meet local needs, training and education, and the building of relationships which are helpful for sustaining and developing practice. There are different ways in which supervision has been developed for complementary therapists in supportive and palliative care settings.
- Individual, with supervisor from the same or different profession
- Small group supervision, with supervisor during work time or in the evening
- Peer supervision, individual or group
- Complementary therapies coordinator supervises own team
- Non-management supervision, such as external supervisor, supervisor from another clinical speciality, complementary therapies coordinator from another centre, perhaps on a mutual exchange basis
- List of supervisors from which the therapist can choose
- Commitment to regular supervision, with agreed contract

## 9.4 Cost of supervision

The cost of supervision may not be an issue for employees who receive in house supervision during work time, but for volunteer and self employed therapists the time and cost involved needs to be considered. Organisations need to be clear within the recruitment process about expectations for the self employed or volunteer therapist to participate in supervision, and about who will meet the costs involved. The sessional payment for self employed therapists could include an element for participation in supervision. Volunteer therapists may consider supervision as part of their support and learning process. Although the process of supervision contributes to quality care, it is against the basic principle of supervision to coerce anyone to participate. Ultimately it is dependent on the creativity and flexibility of provision, as well as the value placed on supervision by therapists.

# 10 Clinical Issues

## 10.1 Introduction

The purpose of this chapter is to give an indication of what therapists can reasonably be expected to know, and the clinical issues in supportive and palliative care of which therapists need to be aware, although there is less emphasis given to neurological conditions than for cancer. These clinical issues fall under three main headings:

- general contraindications and precautions
- issues which patients with cancer may be facing
- issues specific to patients with motor neurone disease, Parkinson's disease and multiple sclerosis

## 10.2 General contraindications and precautions

Therapists trained to the standard required for registration with professional complementary therapy bodies should be knowledgeable about the general contraindications and precautions for the therapy they practise. However, in order to be able to assess the patient prior to treatment, the therapist will need access to the person's medical notes or information about the patient's medical condition(s) and current medication. The latter can be obtained from the patient or via referral forms (See Chapter 11 on referral and assessment and Appendix I).

Staff in conventional healthcare who are not therapists will need familiarisation, guidance or training on:

- when, and when not, to refer patients for complementary therapies.
- how to communicate with patients about complementary therapies, so as not to raise false hopes.

## 10.3 Issues which patients with cancer may be facing

Complementary therapists will need induction and training on the issues which cancer patients may be facing and how these could impact on complementary therapy treatment. The areas for training will depend on the therapist's experience and background. Therapists should have a basic understanding of the conventional treatments patients are likely to receive, how the treatments work and what they are trying to achieve, in order to avoid making uninformed or insensitive comments about the treatment, which can be confusing and distressing for the patient. Therapists need to know

that patients respond as individuals, that the person's condition will fluctuate, and that they may experience different problems and/or emotions at different times. Following are some examples of issues which patients with cancer may be facing.

### A. Issues pre and post diagnosis

**Physical**
- Symptoms depending on the site of the cancer, for example pain or change in body functions
- Symptoms relating to side effects of treatment

**Psycho-spiritual**
- Waiting for results
- Shock, numbness, fear, anxiety, anger, 'why me?'
- Denial
- Living with uncertainty: many aspects of the future, inability to plan; 'how do I cope?'
- Fears about untouchability and infectivity
- Low self-esteem

**Treatment options**
- Surgery
- Radiotherapy
- Chemotherapy
- Hormonal treatment
- Novel therapies, multimodal therapy, etc.
- Clinical trials

**Social**
- In relation to job, family and other relationships
- Isolation, 'who can I talk to?', 'where can I get help?'

### B. Issues relating to treatment

Issues which may be common to all patients include waiting for results and altered body image.

**Surgery**
- Anticipatory fears
- Recovery and convalescence – care needs, wounds, pain and discomfort
- Colostomy and other stoma bags

**Chemotherapy**
- Fatigue
- Discomfort and feeling unwell generally
- Nausea and vomiting
- Hair loss
- Sore mouth and mouth ulcers
- Effects of neutropenia: greater risk of infection, for example, thrush
- Possibility of blood clotting impairment during cycles of chemotherapy
- Diarrhoea
- Altered sensations in extremities
- Altered taste
  See Chapters 12-17 about therapies

**Radiotherapy**
- Fatigue
- Discomfort

- Change in body functions, depending on radiotherapy sites
- Skin sensitivities
- Nausea and vomiting
- Mouth soreness and swallowing difficulties (head and neck treatment)

See Chapters 12-17 about therapies

## Hormonal treatment
- Side effects, such as hot flushes

## Systemic steroids
- Thin skin
- Weakness of thigh and upper arm muscles
- Sleep disturbance
- Altered behaviour or personality

## C. Issues of patients with advanced cancer
It is important to remember that patients have good days too!

### Physical
- Fatigue: their system may be unable to cope with vigorous treatment
- Pain, cancer and non-cancer related
- Increased incidence of undiagnosed deep vein thrombosis as immobility increases
- Discomfort, general and specific areas
- Reduced function of organs or systems leading to, for example, oedema or skin breakdown
- Pathological fractures, if there are bony metastases, or multiple secondaries
- Confusion or disorientation, if there are brain tumours
- Condition can fluctuate greatly

### Emotional
- Anxiety, fear, panic attacks
- Low mood, clinical depression
- Anger, irritation, frustration
- Denial
- Altered body image
- Moods can fluctuate

### Spiritual
- Guilt
- Hopelessness, loss of meaning, faith
- When all active treatment has been discontinued, and the patient is aware that they are dying

### Social
- Plans in relation to family, will, funeral
- Change in personality
- Family dynamics, relationships, problems
- Need for care and support
- Carer's needs
- Financial

### Death
- A patient may die while a therapist is with them (rare)

## D. Therapists need to know what could happen to a patient during a treatment session, albeit rarely
Instructions on what to do in the event of the following:
- Seizure or epileptic fit, usually associated with brain tumours
- Haemorrhage (rare), could be from the stomach via the mouth, the lungs via coughing or via the rectum
- Breathlessness
- Vomiting
- Pain
- Pathological fracture (rare), usually associated with bony metastases

## E. Other important clinical issues
### Deep vein thrombosis (DVT)
- a patient with recent or current DVT should not receive massage to the affected limb.
- a gentle treatment is indicated for patients with advanced cancer as there is a known high incidence of undiagnosed DVT in hospice patients and those with increasing immobility

### Cord compression
- recent loss of skin sensation and/or muscle power in the lower limbs which could indicate compression of the spinal cord

### Intestinal obstruction
- abdominal massage and other treatments that attempt to treat constipation should be avoided unless it is known that the patient is not suffering from intestinal obstruction

### Any change in condition
- the importance of the interprofessional communication role that therapists can have
- who to notify/inform about the patient's change in condition (if relevant)
- what discussion to have with patients who report a change in condition and what advice to give

## 10.4 Issues specific to patients with motor neurone disease, Parkinson's disease or multiple sclerosis

Complementary therapists should be familiarised with the clinical issues with which they may be faced when treating a person with motor neurone disease (MND), Parkinson's disease (PD), and multiple sclerosis (MS) and should be aware of the patient's special needs. The clinical issues that need to be considered include those in Table 2. Further advice and information on neurological diseases can be obtained from:

- The National Hospital for Neurology and Neurosurgery
- Motor Neurone Disease Association
- Multiple Sclerosis Society
- Parkinson's Disease Society
- The department of neurology in local NHS hospital trusts

**Table 2** Clinical issues in motor neurone disease (MND), Parkinson's disease (PD) and multiple sclerosis (MS)

(The presence of the following signs and symptoms depends on the severity of the patient's condition)

| Clinical issue | MND | PD | MS | How this may influence treatment and relationship |
|---|---|---|---|---|
| Level of function impaired | √ | √ on/off | √ | Check with patient, family or nursing staff |
| Moving and handling needs and preferences | √ | √ | √ | Assess, check with patient, family or nursing staff |
| Joint problems or contractures | √ | | √ | May affect moving and handling, check with staff |
| Breathing problems | √ | | | Check with patient, family or staff and position as required |
| Speech impairment | √ | √ | √ | Communication |
| Dribbling of saliva | √ | √ | √ | Assistance with wiping the saliva |
| Difficulty swallowing | √ | √ on/off | √ | |
| Choking attacks | √ | √ on/off | √ | Assist patient and keep calm, summon help as needed |
| Tremor | | √ | | Gentle treatment |
| Rigidity | | √ | | Gentle treatment |
| Spasms, rigidity and pain | √ | | √ | Gentle treatment |
| | | Massage can provoke or increase spasm | | |
| Pain | √ | √ | √ | Gentle treatment |
| | | | Neuropathic | |
| Bradykinesia (slowness) | | √ | | Allow time to relate at the patient's pace |
| Fatigue | √ | | √ | Gentle treatment |
| Oedema in limbs | √ | | √ | |
| Incidence of DVT in advanced disease (depends on level of immobility) | √ | √ | √ | Check with staff |
| Urinary catheter | √ | | √ | |
| PEG feed (feeding tube in abdomen) | √ | | √ | |

Treatment - know what the patient can tolerate, otherwise give only gentle treatments

# 11 Referral and Assessment

## 11.1 Introduction

The referral of patients for complementary therapy treatment relies on a number of factors, including the availability of information for patients, carers and professional staff, healthcare professionals' knowledge of complementary therapies and the resources available within a service. Patients should be given information on the availability of complementary therapy services, and how to access them. (NICE 2002) Assessment of patients prior to treatment also takes different forms and is dependent on a number of factors. This chapter outlines the reasons for which a patient may be referred, the different ways a patient may be referred and assessed, and the documentation involved.

## 11.2 Referral

It is recommended that patients and carers are able to self refer for assessment for complementary therapies. The different routes of referrals are as follows:
* self referral or introduction
* by a family member
* by a health professional

Referral criteria are useful in organisations where health professionals make referrals for complementary therapy treatment, and where responsibility for the patient's care is ultimately the responsibility of the medical team. In these organisations, there will also need to be a system to ensure consent for treatment is obtained or agreed by the relevant medical practitioner. The evidence in the chapters on individual therapies suggests that possible reasons for referral include the following:

* For relaxation
* To improve quality of life through comfort, well being, support
* Tension, stress
* Anxiety, fear, panic attacks
* Low mood, depression
* Pain
* Musculoskeletal problems
* Breathlessness
* Nausea and vomiting
* Constipation
* Hot flushes
* Sleeplessness
* Fatigue
* Body image changes

Patients and carers should be given information leaflets about the different therapies available either within the organisation, or in the local area, in order to facilitate self referral. It is also recommended that professionals are familiarised or trained to routinely discuss the opportunity for complementary therapy treatments with patients and carers. Ideally, patient referrals from professionals should be accompanied by a referral form, which should give the following information:

* Name and date of birth
* Contact information
* Diagnosis: primary and/or secondary cancer sites, Parkinson's disease, multiple sclerosis, motor neurone disease, and year(s) of diagnosis
* Other medical diagnosis
* Current medication
* Details of current chemotherapy treatment (if any) for cancer patients
* Details of current or recent radiotherapy (if any) for cancer patients
* Patient's awareness of diagnosis and prognosis
* Reasons for referral
* Physical symptoms, eg pain, nausea/vomiting, open wounds/lesions, breathlessness, sleeplessness, lymphoedema, DVT
* Other relevant/useful information

An example of a referral form can be seen in Appendix I. However, forms should not inhibit referrals and it may be more appropriate, especially in some circumstances where medical notes are available to the therapist, that the referral is verbal. Where a patient or carer self refers in a non clinical environment, there may not be a referral form, and it is incumbent on the assessor and/or therapist to screen for contraindications or perform a full assessment.

## 11.3 Assessment

The world of complementary therapy can be daunting and an unknown quantity for patients for whom it is new. Patients need to have an explanation (in lay terms) of what the therapies are, what they mean, what is involved in the treatment and what outcome can be hoped for. Leaflets may be available, but should not take the place of discussion, wherever this is possible.

Depending on the setting in which the therapy is provided, the time available and/or the skills of the practitioner, the level of assessment will range from screening for contraindications to a full assessment. Assessment requires the recognition or knowledge of contraindications, change of circumstances and indications of when to discontinue therapy. Contraindications and precautions for use of individual therapies in palliative care can be found in chapters 13-17.

### Screening

Some organisations may decide on a model of service provision in which patients are screened for contraindications. When complementary therapy treatment, usually the touch therapies, is provided in some environments, it may be appropriate for the therapist to carry out a screening for contraindications, rather than a full assessment. These environments include:

- an outpatient environment where the patient may be awaiting or receiving chemotherapy in a room shared with other patients
- an inpatient setting where the room is shared with other patients

### Full assessment

Full assessment includes assessment of physical symptoms, as well as psychological, emotional, social and spiritual factors which have an impact on the patient's life. This form of assessment is likely to elicit information that informs the treatment, but must also be received in a responsible manner (see Chapter 9 on supervision). At some centres, it is the complementary therapy coordinator or team leader who conducts the full assessment. The following issues should be considered prior to a full assessment:

- In an environment where other members of the multidisciplinary team may have carried out a full assessment, the patient's notes should be available to the therapist, in order to avoid duplication. Similarly, a summary of assessments and treatments prescribed, for instance by homeopaths and acupuncturists, should be available for other members of the multidisciplinary team. In service settings where the patient's medical notes are not usually available, the assessor will be able to complete their own assessment.
- The therapist should have had training which enables them to appropriately support the patient through any distressing emotions, without distancing themselves (Heaven & Maguire 1997:A12; Maguire et al 1993)
- The therapist should be aware of other avenues of support to which the patient can be referred
- Supervision should be available to the therapist (refer to Chapter 9 on supervision)

### Key worker assessment

At some centres which offer a wide range of therapies, it may be that designated key workers, who follow the patient's pathway of care through the organisation and who have had specialist assessment training, perform the assessment and decide (with the patient) on the most appropriate course of therapy. In this case:

- The assessment, or a summary, should be available to all the therapists who will be treating the patient.
- The therapist should then make the appropriate

assessment for the therapy provided. Examples of key worker assessment forms can be found in Appendices J and K.

### Communication skills

Communication skills are key to the delivery of effective supportive and palliative care services. (NICE 2002) Specialist assessment and communication skills training is available, and the components of courses which lead to positive outcomes have been identified by NICE (2002) (see Chapter 9.3) Courses currently available include training with:

- Prof. Peter Maguire and team, Psychological Medicine Group, Christie Hospital NHS Trust, Wilmslow Road, Manchester M20 4BX. Tel. 0161 446 3679
- Help the Hospices, Hospice House, 34-44 Britannia Street, London WC1X 9JG. Tel. 020 7520 8200
- St. Ann's Hospice, Institute for Learning and Development, St. Ann's Road North, Heald Green, Cheadle, Cheshire SK8 3SZ. Tel. 0161 437 8136. Contact Christine Lawther, Head of the Institute for Education and Development

## 11.4 Treatment record

Documentation of treatment is an essential element of ethical practice. The following are basic rules for documentation:

- Patient's name and date of birth/hospital/hospice number should be on each page
- Each entry should be signed and dated. Signatures should be identifiable, or a separate record kept to match signatures to individual practitioners.
- The record of treatment should be written legibly
- Entries should be made in ink which allows the document to be legible when photocopied

Examples of treatment records can be seen in Appendix L.

## 11.5 Review of patient and treatment

Different models of practice exist, depending on the organisation and the configuration of the complementary therapy team (see Chapter 3 and Appendix A). With the exception of one-off treatments, it is recommended that there should be a review with the patient, in order to shape and plan further treatments. Reviews may be incorporated into a treatment session, but there should also be periodic reviews with a patient to establish

- Patients' views and level of satisfaction
- The effects, if any, of treatment
- The possibility of treatment with a different therapy

There is advantage in the on-going review being undertaken by a professional other than the therapist(s), but it is important that this person is trained in assessment/review and familiar with complementary therapies. Appendices K and L(i) are examples of practices which incorporate a review of treatment.

# 12 Complementary Therapies

## 12.1 Introduction

This chapter outlines the criteria used for determining the choice of the nine therapies included in the guidelines, the information contained in the chapters which follow on the individual therapies and the methodology used to search for the evidence for each therapy. There are a number of other therapies which are used in supportive and palliative care (Macmillan 2002), but it was not within the resources of this project to include them all.

## 12.2 Criteria for inclusion of therapies in these guidelines

The choice of which therapies to include was guided by:
a. How commonly the therapy is provided in supportive and palliative care services
b. Which therapies are used by conventional medical practitioners and other professionals
c. The existence of professional bodies and regulation for the therapy

Where there are significant similarities for use within supportive and palliative care, the therapies have been grouped, and the nine therapies are:
* touch therapies: aromatherapy, massage and reflexology
* healing/energy therapies: reiki, spiritual healing and therapeutic touch
* hypnosis/hypnotherapy
* acupuncture
* homeopathy

## 12.3 Information provided about each therapy

A brief description of the therapy is followed by information about the evidence base and guidance for the use of the therapy in supportive and palliative care, including conditions for which the therapies may be helpful and contraindications and precautions. Also included is information about the regulation and training of practitioners in that therapy. (See also Chapter 5)

## 12.4 Methodology for reviewing the evidence base

The evidence base for complementary therapies is a significant consideration for managers and clinicians, as well as commissioners and providers of care. However, there is often a misunderstanding of evidence based practice. Evidence based care is described as the conscientious, explicit, and judicious use of current best evidence in making decisions about the care of individual patients. (Sackett 1996) It requires practitioners to integrate the best external evidence with their own clinical expertise and the patient's choice (Sackett 1996).

It is with the above understanding of evidence based practice that these guidelines have been written. It is advisable that the information given about the nine therapies is integrated with the individual practitioner's clinical expertise in deciding whether and how it is appropriate for the patient's clinical state, predicament, and preferences, and whether and how it should be applied.

The search for evidence on the use of the different therapies in palliative care was via the following databases: AMED, BNI, RCN Journals, CINAHL, CISCOM, Medline, PubMed and the databases at the King's Fund. The terms used in the search were: (acupuncture or aromatherapy or massage or reflexology or homeopathy or homoeopathy or acupressure or hypnotherapy or healing or therapeutic touch or reiki) and (pain or anxiety or depression or well-being or well being or constipation or nausea or vomiting or sleep or symptom control or quality of life or self-esteem or self esteem or confidence or mood* or breathlessness or dyspnoea or dyspnea or fatigue or spiritual distress or support or pleasure) and (end of life or palliative care or terminal or hospice or supportive or oncology or cancer or neoplasm or chemotherapy or radiotherapy) and (clinical or trial* or controlled or randomised or non-randomised or systematic review* or qualitative or study or research or project or audit or evaluation or pilot or patient* survey* or consumer choice).

The purpose of the above was to search for evidence on how the therapies may be useful in cancer and palliative care. It was not the intention of the project, nor within its scope, to conduct a systematic review of evidence and this was not performed. Evidence was also identified through collaboration with colleagues in the different fields and the sharing of information.

The available literature was sorted and reviewed according to the following categories wherever possible and a summary is provided of symptoms and conditions with which the therapy may be useful in supportive and palliative care.

- Evidence derived from randomised controlled trials or reviews of randomised trials
- Evidence from prospective studies with a comparison group (non-randomised controlled study or observational studies)
- Comparison groups, calculation of sample size and accurate, standard definition of outcome variables
- Cross-sectional studies
- Professional consensus

# 13 Touch Therapies

## 13.1 Introduction

This chapter gives guidance on the use of the three touch therapies most commonly provided within supportive and palliative care: massage, aromatherapy, and reflexology. These therapies have been grouped together because the conditions in which they may be helpful, and the precautions for their use, are similar. Information is included on whether massage spreads cancer, as this seems to be a question that is frequently raised. The control of infection is an issue for all therapies, but particularly so for the touch therapies; the principles of universal infection control are outlined.

## 13.2 Use of touch therapies in supportive and palliative care

The areas common to massage, aromatherapy and reflexology are described first, followed separately by descriptions of and the evidence base for each therapy.

### When touch therapies may be helpful
The best available evidence suggests that massage, aromatherapy and reflexology may be useful in the following ways:

- **To promote relaxation** (Ferrell-Torry & Glick 1992, Dossey et al 1995, Corner et al 1995, Van de Riet 1999, Byass 1999, Hodgson 2000, Wilkie et al 2000, Manasse 2001, Hadfield 2001, Grealish 2002, Gambles, Crooke & Wilkinson 2002)
- **To alleviate anxiety** (Ferrell-Torry & Glick 1992, Corner et al 1995, Wilkinson et al 1999, Byass 1999, Stephenson et al 1999, Hills & Taylor 2001, Gambles, Crooke & Wilkinson 2002)
- **To reduce depression** (Wilkinson 1995, Field 1998, Hills & Taylor 2001, Jorm et al 2002)
- **To reduce pain** (Ferrell-Torry & Glick 1992, Smith et al 1994, Wilkinson 1995, Field 1998, Byass 1999, Van der Riet 1999, Wilkie et al 2000, Grealish et al 2002)
- **To reduce nausea** (Grealish et al 2002)
- **To alleviate symptoms**, such as breathlessness, constipation, diarrhoea, pain, nausea, fatigue, poor appetite (for reflexology: Hodgson 2000, Hills & Taylor 2001)
- **To alleviate side effects of chemotherapy** (for reflexology: Hills & Taylor 2001)
- **To improve sleep pattern** (Hills & Taylor 2001)
- **To reduce stress and tension** (Garnett 1994, Wilkinson 1995, Dossey et al 1995, Micozzi 1996)
- **To reduce psychological distress/provide**

emotional support (Trousdall 1996, Kite, Maher et al 1998, Hodgson 2000, Hills & Taylor 2001)
- **To improve well-being and quality of life** (Wilkinson 1995, Wilkie et al 2000, Hodgson 2000, Hills & Taylor 2001, Billhult & Dahlberg 2001)
- **To live with an altered body image** (Bredin 1999, Van der Riet 1999)

### Does massage spread cancer?
This is a question that is frequently raised and an area where there is some confusion. Gentle massage can be given to areas of the body not affected by cancer. Some oncologists and radiotherapists have stated that there is no evidence that massage increases the spread of lymphoma or indeed leukaemia cells, and that cancer is not a contraindication to receiving gentle massage (Sikora 1991, cited McNamarra 1999). MacDonald (1999) describes how cancer spreads, directly and indirectly. Cancer spreads even while patients are resting and inactive, for instance sleeping or just sitting. Gentle massage does not increase vascular or lymphatic circulation any more than the activities of daily living, such as exercise, shopping, taking a warm bath (MacDonald 1999).

Massage therapists are advised to be cautious over tumour sites, because any mechanical force on the tumour may contribute to the pressure already taking place due to the uncontrolled growth of the cancer, and may influence spread. Deep massage to any part of the body is not advisable for those with active cancer, in order to avoid trauma and activation of the immune response (MacDonald 1999). It is also advisable for therapists to work within the boundaries of current contraindications and precautions for supportive and palliative care.

### General contraindications
Massage therapists, aromatherapists and reflexologists are trained to assess and screen for conditions in which treatment is contraindicated for any individual, for instance when the person is pyrexial.

### Precautions
Therapists with limited experience will need further training and/or supervision (see Chapter 9 on supervision) from therapists experienced in the use of the therapy in supportive and palliative care. Clinical issues to be considered for people with motor neurone disease, Parkinson's disease and multiple sclerosis are addressed in Chapter 10. The following guidelines on the use of aromatherapy, massage and reflexology in cancer care form a general consensus amongst complementary therapy practitioners in cancer and palliative care (McNamarra 1999, Hodkinson & Williams 2002), and should be included in induction and training, as needed.

a) Aromatherapy and massage
- **Avoid** using any pressure directly on the area of the cancer
- **Avoid** pressure work with patients who are taking anti-coagulation medication or who have a low platelet count. What is considered a low platelet count varies; some haematologists advise that patients with a platelet count of 50,000 or less are not treated with massage or aromatherapy.
- **Be aware** of the risks of massaging patients with areas of petechiae (pinprick bruising is an indicator of very low platelet count). Use gentle stroking or light, holding touch only, unless working in a specialist area and in consultation with the medical team.
- **Avoid** a limb or foot with suspected or recently diagnosed deep vein thrombosis. Check with clinical team, be aware of signs and symptoms of deep vein thrombosis.
- **Be aware** that patients with advanced cancer or severely impaired mobility are more susceptible to low grade, undiagnosed and asymptomatic deep vein thrombosis (Johnson et al 1999); use gentle massage only
- **Avoid** areas of bony metastases, and use gentle stroking or light, holding touch only
- **Only treat** lymphoedematous limbs or areas if working in conjunction with a lymphoedema specialist nurse or physiotherapist. In the absence of specialists, refer to local policy or avoid working the area or limb.
- **Avoid** massaging over ascites (fluid retention in the abdomen) and use gentle stroking or light holding touch only
- **Avoid** stoma sites, dressings, catheters and TENS machines.
- **Be aware** that patients have a lowered immune function and are more susceptible to infection
- **Be aware** that the skin can be sensitive, and/or paper thin due to medication and treatment, especially in elderly or cachectic patients. Use gentle touch only.
- **Be aware** of other clinical issues (See Chapter 10)
- Radiotherapy
  **Be aware** of possible side effects, such as fatigue, soreness of skin, digestive disturbance
  **Avoid** the entry and exit sites during and for 3-6 weeks following radiotherapy; check with patient and assess whether the skin is still sensitive, tender or sore
  **Encourage** the patient to seek advice from the radiotherapy department regarding the use of gels and creams
- Chemotherapy
  **Be aware** of possible side effects of chemotherapy on the whole person, for instance extreme fatigue, lowered immune function and increased risk of infection, increased risk of bruising, dryness or peeling of skin, digestive disturbance, nausea, altered

sensation in extremities, hair loss, altered behaviour or personality, skin sensitive to touch
  **Be aware** that patients could have altered smell preferences
  **Consider** using gentle massage only, as the patient may not be able to cope with even moderately energising or vigorous treatment
- **Modify** pressure and adapt approach and duration of session to take account of the patient's preference, and also the physical, emotional and energetic condition of the patient. For instance use gentle stroking or light touch if the patient is very tired, unwell or emotionally labile. Be guided by the patient's body language and clinical issues (see Chapter 10).
- **Consider** massaging part of the body only and in shorter sessions.
- **Use of essential oils** is addressed separately in the section on aromatherapy (13.4).
- **Aromatherapy via vapourisers**
  **Be aware** of respiratory conditions such as asthma
  **Be aware** when used in a room where there are other patients or individuals with respiratory conditions, or different smell preferences or allergies
  **Use electric vapourisers** in the presence of oxygen
  **Use burners with caution**: follow the health and safety policy of the organisation with regards to risk of fire if using aromatherapy burners, for instance patients should not be left on their own at any time when a burner is used and burners should not be left unattended.

b) Reflexology
- **Avoid** a limb or foot with suspected deep vein thrombosis and avoid varicose veins.
- **Be aware** of any tender areas on the foot or hand that relate to new surgical wounds.
- **Only treat** lymphoedematous limbs or areas, if working in conjunction with a lymphoedema specialist. In the absence of a specialist, refer to local policy or avoid working the area or limb.
- **Avoid** areas corresponding to colonic stimulation if there are any symptoms or risk of intestinal obstruction due to causes other than constipation.
- **Adjust** pressure for patients with a low platelet count, taking note of any existing bruising and skin viability. What is considered a low platelet count varies; some haematologists advise that patients with a platelet count of 50,000 or less are not treated with reflexology.
- **Be aware** that peripheral sensation may be affected by a person's psychological state, or medication, such as steroids, opioids or chemotherapy.
- **Be aware** that peripheral neuropathy may be a symptom of diseases such as multiple sclerosis and certain tumours, although diabetes is the most common cause of peripheral neuropathy.

- **Palpate gently** and sensitively over the reflexes relating to tumour site(s)
- **Assess the condition** of the reflexes and adapt treatment accordingly so that the feet are not overstimulated in any way, especially in patients with altered peripheral sensation or peripheral neuropathy
- **Establish** a working pressure that is comfortable for the patient at all times, and tailor treatment to avoid strong reactions
- **Use** fragrance free talcum powder or appropriate cream if the skin is very dry

### Teaching carers/patients

It may be helpful to the patient and/or their carers for the therapist to teach them basic massage skills, with or without essential oils.

### Side effects and adverse effects

Complementary therapists should discuss possible side effects which should not be a cause for concern with patients, for instance that they may feel drowsy following treatment and want to sleep. Possible reactions to essential oils are addressed in the section on aromatherapy (see 13.4).

### Infection control

Universal infection control procedures are precautions to be followed at all times to prevent the spread of infection, as it is not always possible to identify people who may spread infection to others. All blood and body fluids are potentially infectious and precautions are necessary to prevent exposure to them. (Department of Health 1996, Mallett & Dougherty 2000) These routine procedures should be familiar to therapists with a conventional healthcare qualification but may not be familiar to others.
- Complementary therapists should follow good basic hygiene practices at all times including thorough hand washing before and after treating a patient.
- If the therapist has any grazes, cuts or any wound in the hands, these areas should be covered with a waterproof dressing. Under health and safety legislation, such dressings must always be available in the first aid box. (Department of Health 1996)
- Therapists with any skin condition on their hands that cannot be covered with a waterproof dressing should seek medical advice and clearance prior to providing hands-on therapies.
- Should the therapist need to deal with spillages of blood, vomit, urine or excreta, a disposable apron and gloves should be worn.
- Methicillin Resistant Staphylococcus Aureus (MRSA) is addressed specifically in these guidelines because of the widespread concern and lack of knowledge on this issue.
  (i) The prevention of spread of MRSA between patients is very much dependent on the proper understanding and practice of universal infection control procedures.

(ii) The single most important practice is proper hand hygiene, before and after attending to the patient. If the patient is isolated in an inpatient unit, there may be additional procedures on leaving the room, such as using an alcoholic or bactericidal hand rub in addition to hand washing procedures inside the room.

(iii) Some organisations with inpatients require therapists to wear gloves and others do not. Therapists will need to check.

(iv) When treating a patient with MRSA in an environment where there are other patients the therapist may be treating, it is generally advised that an apron is worn.
- Training and guidance on infection control should be considered within the induction programme for new therapists.

### Regulation and training of therapists

Training in massage, aromatherapy and reflexology is currently available in a large number of schools and institutions, privately as well as in community and further education colleges and universities. Courses vary in length, depth and quality. A guide to choosing complementary therapy courses is published by The Prince of Wales's Foundation for Integrated Health (Williams 2003).

For further information please see Chapter 5 on regulation and training, Chapter 6 about recruitment and selection and Chapter 7 on volunteers.

## 13.3 Massage

### Brief description

Massage is a generic term for a variety of techniques that involve touching, pressing, kneading, and manipulation of the soft tissues of the body for therapeutic purposes (Calvert 1992; Jackson 1993). There are a number of types of massage, (Russell 1994) for example Swedish, Thai, Ayurvedic, remedial, and sports massage. The precise method depends on the culture from which the technique originated, and the philosophy on which it is based. Individual practitioners are likely to have developed a particular style, based on their skills, interest, philosophy and experience with different client groups.

Massage therapy in supportive and palliative care refers to therapeutic massage, in which touch is considered to be an independent channel of communication. (Weiss 1979, Westland 1993, McNamara 1999) The essence of the therapeutic process is embodied in the concepts of skilful touch, (Juhan 1987) and essential touch. (Smith 1990)

In cancer care, Simonton (1991, cited McNamarra 1999:21) indicates that "good therapeutic massage is massage done by a well-trained massage therapist who is sensitive to the problems of massaging people with cancer, and is comfortable dealing with people who are seriously ill." Therapeutic massage consists of gentle rhythmical touch, with movements varied to suit individual needs and with a clear start and finish to the session. (McNamara 1999)

The recognition that touch and massage can have therapeutic value dates back to the *Yellow Emperor's Classic of Internal Medicine* (about 250 BC), Sanskrit texts, Homer's Odyssey, Hippocrates and Asclepiades, Galen in the Middle Ages, and Paracelsus in the 15-16th centuries. There is a vast amount of anecdotal as well as research evidence which suggests that massage therapy has the potential to produce physiological and psychological benefits for palliative care patients (cited Wilkie et al 2000). There are many theories about how massage works; see for instance Juhan 1987 and McNamara 1999.

### Evidence base

In cancer care, the scientific evidence relies on a number of studies, mainly based on small numbers. Corner et al's (1995) quasi-experimental study with 52 cancer patients over 8 weeks found that massage had a significant effect on anxiety, assisted relaxation and reduced physical and emotional symptoms. Wilkie et al (2000) carried out a randomised controlled pilot study with 29 patients to evaluate the effects of massage on pain intensity, analgesics and quality of life of cancer patients. The study confirmed the findings of other studies, that the use of massage to modify anxiety and the perception of cancer pain is effective in the short-term. (Ferrell-Torry & Glick 1992; Meek 1993, Weinrich & Weinrich 1990)

The results from Wilkinson et al's (1999) study with 103 cancer patients, randomised to receive massage or aromatherapy, suggest that massage, either with or without an essential oil, is beneficial for reducing anxiety levels in patients with advanced cancer. Grealish et al (2000) measured the short term effects of foot massage on pain, nausea and relaxation in 87 hospitalised cancer patients, using a quasi-experimental research design. Foot massage was found to have a significant immediate effect on reducing pain and nausea, and encouraging relaxation.

Pan et al's (2000) systematic review of complementary and alternative medicine in the management of pain, dyspnoea and nausea and vomiting near the end of life concludes that, amongst other therapies, massage may provide pain relief.

A Cochrane Review taking forward the work of Cooke & Ernst (2000) is in process, to review the use of aromatherapy and massage for symptom relief in patients with cancer. The objective is to assess the evidence for the effectiveness of aromatherapy and/or massage in improving physical and psychological well-being in patients with cancer. (Fellowes, Barnes & Wilkinson 2003) 1323 references were retrieved. Nine met the inclusion criteria and a further two are still under consideration. The nine that met the inclusion criteria included references representing seven studies, all of which were randomised controlled trials. Assimilation of results from the seven trials, and consideration of two new studies is ongoing. Initial trends suggest that massage confers some short-term benefits over no massage, and aromatherapy massage confers some additional benefit when compared with non-aromatherapy massage. Studies have measured changes in a range of physical and psychological symptoms, and in quality of life measures, but sample sizes were small and in most cases follow-up times were short.

Billhult and Dahlberg's (2001) phenomenological research on eight female cancer patients' experience of massage on 10 consecutive days, describes the experience of 'meaningful relief'. The relief was meaningful for a number of reasons: it offered relief from suffering, an experience of being able to 'feel good' in spite of the cancer and its treatment, feeling 'special', empowerment and autonomy, and the massage contributed to the development of a positive relationship with the therapist.

Bredin (1999) conducted a qualitative study of three women's experience of therapeutic massage following mastectomy and body image problems. She concluded that therapeutic massage, combined with listening to the women's experiences, could help with certain aspects of adjustment to having had a mastectomy.

Audits and evaluations of service and interviews show that patients feel they benefit from massage (for example Bell 1999; Billhult & Dahlberg 2001; Byass 1999; Wilkinson 1995). Patients seek therapies to enhance hope, (Downer et al 1994) as well as to reduce anxiety, stress and pain. The evidence of use clearly shows that massage is one of most widely-used therapies in supportive and palliative care (Wilkes 1992; Ernst 1997; Coss 1998; Bell 1999; Foundation for Integrated Medicine, 2001; Lewith et al 2001; MacMillan 2002).

It may be concluded that massage is an acceptable intervention with cancer patients.

## 13.4 Aromatherapy

### Brief description

Aromatherapy is the systematic use of essential oils in treatments to improve physical and emotional well-being. (*National Occupational Standards for Aromatherapy,* Healthwork UK 2002) Many plant species contain essential oils, highly fragrant and flammable essences, which evaporate quickly and which are extracted from plants by a distillation process. (Tisserand 1988) Aromatherapists in the U.K. are trained to use essential oils topically and through inhalation. (Buckle 1997) Essential oils are applied in a variety of ways, which include massage, vapourisers, baths, creams and lotions, and compresses, and are absorbed through the skin, diluted in a vegetable carrier oil or by inhalation.

Essential oils have been used in many cultures throughout history. Aromatherapy as we now know it, owes its development and name to Rene-Maurice Gattefosse, a French chemist, who was impressed by the healing powers of lavender essential oil on burns and began to study the healing powers of essential oils in the early 20th century. Elsewhere in the European Union essential oils can be taken orally when prescribed by medical doctors and medical herbalists trained in their use.

The therapeutic effect of aromatherapy results from a combination of the physiological effects of the oils and the relaxation of massage. As the fragrance of the oils also stimulates the sense of smell, which elicits certain emotions, the limbic system of the midbrain, which is concerned with emotional as well as visceral function, may be involved in the release of hormones which influence mood. (Kohn 1999)

### Evidence base

As massage is the most widely used medium for applying essentials oils in palliative care, the evidence for massage therapy (see 13.3) should be considered with this section .

Cooke & Ernst (2000) undertook a systematic review of the use of essential oils and aromatherapy massage in reducing anxiety for patients in a health care setting. Six trials met the inclusion criteria. Three studies were conducted in cancer and palliative care, evaluating the use of aromatherapy and essential oils with massage for reduction of anxiety and symptom scores, and increase in well-being and quality of life. (Corner et al 1995; Wilkinson 1995; Wilkinson et al 1999) The results of the studies suggest that aromatherapy massage can be helpful for anxiety reduction in the short term.

However Cooke & Ernst (2000) concluded that the trials were comprised of small samples and lacked methodological rigour. There was no differentiation between the effects of any transdermal absorption, the effects of smell and the influence of psychological factors. The methodologies were considered "sufficiently flawed to prevent firm conclusions from being drawn". However, it was acknowledged that a double-blind design to compare

aromatherapy treatments is probably impossible to achieve. In view of the above, and the increasing popularity of aromatherapy, it was recommended that national guidelines on the use of aromatherapy (and other complementary therapies) within the health service should be developed.

Corner et al's (1995) quasi-experimental study with 52 cancer patients, compared the effect of an eight week course of massage, with or without a blend of essential oils, on patients undergoing cancer treatment. Patients were randomised into one of two treatment groups, with a control group of patients who were unable to attend for massage. Patients were interviewed before the study began and at eight weeks following completion, and outcome measures included the Hospital Anxiety and Depression scale (Zigmond and Snaith 1983) and a quality of life and symptom distress scale (Holmes and Dickerson 1987). The results suggest that massage has an effect on anxiety, and this was found to be greater where essential oils were used. Massage also assisted relaxation and significantly improved emotional symptoms, in particular concentration, mood and feelings about appearance and the future. Massage with essential oils showed overall improvement in pain, mobility, tiredness, function and ability to return to paid employment.

Wilkinson et al (1999) researched the effectiveness of massage and aromatherapy massage in improving the quality of life of patients with advanced cancer, and patients' perception of the value of aromatherapy massage in improving their quality of life. Patients were randomly allocated to one of two treatment groups, and received a course of three full body massages, with or without the essential oil Roman camomile. Outcome measurements included the Rotterdam Symptom Checklist (De Haes et al 1990), the State-Trait Anxiety Inventory (Spielberger et al 1983), and a semi-structured questionnaire completed 2 weeks after the last treatment to explore patients' perceptions of the treatment. Both the preliminary study with 51 patients (Wilkinson 1995) and the final results with 103 patients (Wilkinson et al 1999) showed an improvement in quality of life in both groups, with statistical significance in the aromatherapy group. The results also showed a significant reduction in anxiety in both groups, although the effect was transient. Comparison of results between the two groups suggests that massage with essential oil enhances the effects of massage, and improves physical and psychological symptoms, as well as overall quality of life. From the patients' perception, massage or aromatherapy is beneficial in reducing anxiety, tension, pain and depression.

A study not included in the Cooke & Ernst (2000) review was a randomised controlled pilot study (Manderson, Weller, Wilcock, Ernst et al 2001) which assessed the effect of aromatherapy massage in palliative day care. Forty-six patients were randomised to receive day care alone or day care plus weekly aromatherapy massage for four weeks, using a standardised blend of oils. Outcome measures included the centre's own questionnaires which rated quality of life, physical symptoms and patient satisfaction. The scale Profile of Mood States (POMS) was also used. All patients were satisfied with aromatherapy massage and wanted to continue with treatment. There was improvement in all measures in both groups but there was no statistically significant difference between the groups. Due to the high attrition rate, it was recommended that multi-centre trials were necessary for studies of sufficient power.

A multi-centre randomised controlled trial (Wilkinson, Ramirez, Maher, Sun, et al 1999) to evaluate the use of aromatherapy massage in improving psychological distress and other components of quality of life in patients with cancer has been designed in line with Cooke & Ernst's (2000) recommendations. The inclusion criterion was patients with cancer who were psychologically distressed, assessed by a structured psychiatric interview as experiencing depression and/or generalised anxiety disorder. Results of this study will be reported in early 2003.

A Cochrane Review to take forward the work of Cooke & Ernst (2000) is in process. The use of aromatherapy and massage for symptom relief in patients with cancer is being reviewed, with the objective of assessing the evidence for the effectiveness of aromatherapy and/or massage in improving physical and psychological well-being in patients with cancer (Fellowes, Barnes & Wilkinson 2003). 1323 references were retrieved. Nine met the inclusion criteria and a further two are still under consideration. The nine that met the inclusion criteria included references representing seven studies, all of which were randomised controlled trials. Assimilation of results from the seven trials, and consideration of two new studies is ongoing. Initial trends suggest that massage confers some short-term benefits over no massage, and aromatherapy massage confers some additional benefit when compared with non-aromatherapy massage. Studies measured changes in a range of physical and psychological symptoms, and in quality of life measures, but sample sizes were small and in most cases follow-up times were short.

There are a number of service evaluations and audits on the use of aromatherapy massage in cancer care. (eg Evans 1995; Kite, Maher et al 1998; de Valois & Clarke 2001, Hills & Taylor 2001; Hadfield 2001) The findings are similar to those of the abovementioned trials, showing improvement in psychological symptoms such as anxiety,

depression, tension, stress, emotions such as fear, anger, guilt, as well as physical symptoms including pain. From the patients' perception, relaxation and reduced tension are most commonly identified benefits.

Despite the lack of scientific evidence on the effects of aromatherapy, it remains one of the most widely used therapies in supportive and palliative care. (Foundation for Integrated Medicine, 2001; Manasse 2001, Lewith et al 2002, Macmillan 2002) From the patients' perspective, the service evaluations and audits also support perceived effectiveness and satisfaction. (Dunwoody, Smyth & Davidson 2002)

### Essential oils

In the absence of scientific data, the following guidelines form a general consensus amongst aromatherapists working in palliative care (eg Buckle 1997; Price & Price 1995; Foundation for Integrated Medicine 2001).

There is a difference in opinion regarding the need to recommend oils which are considered safe and those to be avoided or used with precaution in certain conditions, such as with oestrogen sensitive cancers, patients with reduced kidney function and hypertension. There is no definitive evidence to support the range of opinions, and it is recommended that professionals refer to the work of Tisserand and Balacs (1995) *Essential Oil Safety*, and to experienced aromatherapists working in supportive and palliative care.

#### a) The decision to use essential oils

- The decision to use and mix essential oils should only be made by aromatherapists who are registered with an appropriate professional body (see Chapter 5 and Appendix E).
- Essential oils should only be used and mixed by aromatherapists following an assessment of the patient or screening for contraindications
- Develop a protocol for the safe use of a range of essential oils by other members of the clinical team in situations such as use with vapourisers
- Massage therapists, practitioners of simple massage or carers who have been shown how to massage the patient should use blends made by aromatherapists for the individual patient

#### b) Blending and strength of oils

- It is the general consensus within aromatherapy education and training that a 1% dilution (or less) is used in massage with children and adults in poor health.
- For the use of essential oils in the bath, it is suggested that the oils should be diluted in a non-oil-based medium (to 1% or less). Oils should not be added undiluted to bath water as they may cause irritation if the patient has sensitive skin. In particular, patients undergoing or having recently

undergone radiotherapy or chemotherapy may have hypersensitive skin.

## c) Buying oils
- Essential oils should be purchased from suppliers who provide a safety data sheet for each oil purchased (CHIP 1994; COSHH 1994; Buckle 1997), including a GLC readout of constituents of the oil.
- There are numerous suppliers of essential oils and the importance of using pure essential oils is stressed in the training of aromatherapists.
- It is suggested that organisations purchase essential oils from suppliers recommended by aromatherapists who provide a service within the organisation.

## d) Storage and packaging
Undiluted essential oils should be stored and packaged as follows. (Buckle 1997; Price & Price 1995; Tisserand & Balacs 1995)
- In a locked container at all times, away from naked flames, food or drink
- Oxidation changes the chemical composition of essential oils, and the process is speeded up by heat and light. Undiluted essential oils should be:
  (i) packaged in blue or amber glass bottles, away from direct sunlight
  (ii) packaged in glass bottles containing integral droppers of UK standard (20 drops per ml).
  (iii) stored in a cool environment
- The bottle should indicate a packaged or use by date.

## e) Accidents with essential oils (Buckle 1997:102)
- Skin reaction to undiluted essential oil
  Dilute with carrier oil (to dilute), then wash the area with unperfumed soap and water and dry. Keep the bottle to show content, and seek medical assistance
- Undiluted essential oil splashed in the eye
  Irrigate the eye with milk or carrier oil (to dilute), and then with water. Keep the bottle to show content, and seek medical assistance
- Ingestion of more than 5 mls of essential oil (to be treated as poisons)
  Give milk to drink, keep the bottle to show content and seek medical assistance.
- Essential oil bottle broken and oil is spilt
  Gloves should be worn to prevent the skin becoming contaminated with the undiluted essential oil. Soak up the liquid with paper towel and collect the glass. Dispose of glass in the sharps container in a clinical environment, or wrap in layers of paper and dispose in secured polythene bag in other settings

## f) Disposal
Empty bottles should be disposed of in a sharps container in a clinical environment, or wrapped in layers of paper and disposed of in a secured polythene bag in other settings

# 13.5 Reflexology

### Brief description
Reflexology is based on the principle that there are reflex areas in the feet and hands which correspond to all of the glands, organs and parts of the body (*National Occupational Standards for Reflexology*, Healthwork UK 2002). The purpose of the systematic application of pressure, using the thumb and fingers, to specific reflex points on the feet or hands is to release congestion, promote the flow of energy and promote homeostasis.

Different types of foot treatment have been used in various cultures including India, Egypt and China since ancient times. In the west, reflexology developed in the 20th century through the discoveries of the American ear, nose and throat specialist, William Fitzgerald, and was further refined by massage therapist, Eunice Ingham. Doreen Bayly brought the treatment to Europe and established the first school of reflexology in the UK. Reflexology, reflex zone therapy or reflexotherapy are all terms that refer to the current use of the treatment, and are associated with developments by individuals such as Hanne Marquardt, Froneberg, and Pat Morrell. (Tiran 2002)

The language of reflexology is not easily understood by people with conventional western medical training. Within conventional health care, reflexology may be more easily understood as a sophisticated system of touch. (Tiran 2002) Techniques include the application of pressure to all areas of the feet or hands that relate to a map of the whole body. Reflexologists claim to feel areas which have an altered granular texture at specific points in the foot, indicative of imbalance, weakness or disease of the corresponding body part and then massage these and other related areas.

Reflexologists do not diagnose specific medical problems, but aim to treat the individual, with a view to alleviating physical and emotional symptoms. (Lynn 1996, *National Occupational Standards for Reflexology*, Healthwork UK 2002).

### Evidence base
A randomised controlled study of reflexology treatments for 35 women with premenstrual syndrome during an eight week period showed a decrease in premenstrual signs and symptoms (including anxiety), significantly more in the intervention group than in the placebo group. (Oleson & Flocco 1993)

Stephenson et al (2000) completed a quasi-experimental crossover study on the effects of foot reflexology on anxiety and pain in 23 patients with breast or lung cancer. A Visual Analogue Scale (Cline, Herman, Shaw & Morton 1992) was used to measure anxiety, and the Short-Form McGill Pain Questionnaire (Melzack 1987) to measure pain. The study reported a significant decrease in anxiety; the effects on pain reduction were less clear.

Foot massage was used as a nursing intervention in a quasi-experimental study with 87 patients hospitalised with cancer. (Grealish et al 2000) Patients were randomly assigned to one of three factor control groups and heart rate was monitored. Visual analogue scales were used to measure self reports of pain, nausea and vomiting, and relaxation. Their findings showed that foot massage has a significant immediate effect on pain, nausea and relaxation.

Hodgson's (2000) study compared the effects of a course of three real or placebo reflexology treatments on the quality of life of 11 patients with cancer. The outcome measures included the Holmes and Dickerson (1987) quality of life scale, modified to incorporate an open-ended question for patients' comments. There was statistical significance in the difference in improvement in quality of life between the two groups. All the patients in the reflexology group reported an improvement. However, improvement in breathing was the only individual symptom with a statistically significant result. The patients' perception, in both groups, was that it was relaxing, calming and comforting.

A Cochrane systematic review on the use of reflexology for symptom relief in patients with cancer is nearing completion. (Fellows, Gambles, Lockhart-Wood, Wilkinson 2003) The objective of this review is to assess the evidence for the effectiveness of reflexology in improving physical and psychological wellbeing in patients with cancer. 312 references were retrieved; only three met the inclusion criteria. The three references represented two randomised controlled trials, both of which have been mentioned above.

Both trials found some positive effects for reflexology. Hodgson (2000) found significant differences between groups for overall scores and for breathing, with greater benefits in the reflexology group. In the Stephenson (2000) crossover trial, anxiety scores were significantly lower after reflexology than after control. Significant improvements in pain scores were found after reflexology and after control. However, the Cochrane review concludes that methodological problems occurred for both trials. Sample sizes were small, and follow up was very limited. Possibility for bias occurred in both studies and no comparisons were possible to determine if repeated treatments confer additional benefits. In addition, neither study sought to record adverse effects so it is not possible to know if any exist.

Audit and evaluation of services similarly identify relaxation, relief from tension and anxiety, and improved well-being as the primary benefits of reflexology in palliative care. (Hills & Taylor 2001; Milligan et al 2002; Gambles, Crooke and Wilkinson 2002)

There is much anecdotal literature which similarly supports the use of reflexology in cancer care for relaxation, wellbeing and stress relief. (Gillard 1995; Stephenson 1996; Botting 1997; Joyce & Richardson 1997; Tanner 2000; Hodkinson 2000). Despite the lack of scientific evidence, surveys of patient use reveal that reflexology is one of the most widely used therapies in cancer care. (Oneschuk et al 2000; Lewith et al 2001; Foundation for IntegratedMedicine 2001; Manasse 2000; Macmillan 2002; Gambles, Crooke & Wilkinson 2002)

# 14 Healing and energy therapies

## 14.1 Introduction

The term healing is from the Saxon root *Haelen*, meaning to make whole and is not seen as a desire to cure or as an attachment to a particular outcome. (Hallett 2002) The term subtle energy techniques is also used in the context of healing. (MacDonald 1999) There are a number of energy therapies and this chapter focuses on the use of reiki, therapeutic touch and spiritual healing as the mostly widely used in palliative care. (Macmillan 2002) The conditions in which these therapies may be helpful, and the precautions for their use are outlined, followed by descriptions, the evidence base and training for each therapy.

## 14.2 The use of healing and energy therapies in supportive and palliative care

The conditions for which reiki, spiritual healing and therapeutic touch may be useful are similar, as are the precautions for the use of these therapies in supportive and palliative care.

### When healing and energy therapies may be useful

The best available evidence suggests that reiki, spiritual healing or therapeutic touch may be useful in the following ways:

- **To contribute to pain relief** (Keller & Bzdek 1986, Gordon et al 1998, Neate & Neate 2001, Benor 2001, Hills & Taylor 2002)
- **To promote relaxation** (Krieger et al 1979, Heidt 1981, Quinn 1982, Wardell & Engerretson 2001, Neate & Neate 2001)
- **To improve sleep pattern** (Braun et al 1986, Hills & Taylor 2003)
- **To reduce tension, stress and anxiety** (Heidt 1981, Quinn 1982, Olsen 1992, Hallett 1996, Neate & Neate 2001, Wardell & Engerretson 2001, Hills & Taylor 2003)
- **To provide emotional and/or spiritual support** (Hallett 1996, Hallett 2000, Neate & Neate 2001, Benor 2001, Hills & Taylor 2002)
- **To contribute to a sense of well being** (Hallett 1996, Hallett 2000, Neate & Neate 2001, Hills & Taylor 2002)
- **To reduce side effects of chemotherapy and radiotherapy** (Neate & Neate 2001)
- **To support the patient in the dying process** (Neate & Neate 2001)

### General contraindications and precautions

There are no specific contraindications, but there are some precautions for the use of healing in supportive and palliative care:

- Give healing treatment only in response to a request from the patient or carer and following consent from the patient.
- Be aware that the patient may misunderstand the word healing to mean cure; emphasise healing may be physical, psychological, emotional or spiritual, but discuss possible benefits in a way that does not raise false hopes. Emphasise that there is no religious association.
- Be sensitive to the needs of the patient, and give healing in a position that is comfortable for the patient, rather than the customary positions of sitting in a chair or lying flat on a couch.
- Use with sensitivity with patients and carers who, because of their personal history, disease progression or medication, may have an altered perception of reality, either emotionally or mentally.
- Be aware that the relaxation response can act as a releasing mechanism, which can sometimes generate strong emotions. It is important that practitioners should be aware of this, and be able to allow and contain strong emotions. Spiritual healers who are undergoing training are known as probationary healers and normally practise healing when a fully qualified healer is available for advice.
- Ensure that sessions are not overlong; an experienced practitioner can generally recognize when healing is completed in a particular session.

### Teaching carers and patients

Reiki is a healing therapy that patient and carers can learn from a reiki master for self treatment and to use with family and friends.

### Infection control

Refer to Chapter 13.2.

### Regulation and Training

For information on the regulation of therapists, refer to Chapter 5. There is information on levels of training for the three healing therapies in the following sections on the individual healing therapies.

## 14.3 Reiki

### Brief description

Reiki is a method of healing that was rediscovered by Dr Mikao Usui in Japan in the 1800s. Central to this system of healing is the concept that an energy flow exists within living beings which supports life by helping to maintain homeostasis. This energy is known as Ki. When Ki is diminished ill health can arise. The other important concept is that Ki can be channelled from its originating source by a reiki practitioner and passed on to a recipient. The original source may be referred to as the universal source, which in Japanese is Rei, hence the name reiki. The main aim of reiki is to bring about balance in mind, body and spirit to improve well-being. There are no religious connotations within reiki, therefore no belief system is necessary to practise or receive this method of healing.

Reiki was primarily developed as a system for healing oneself, as well as being used to help others, therefore practitioners are encouraged to practise self-healing on a regular basis. A reiki treatment, for oneself or another, involves the practitioner placing his/her hands either on, or just above, certain points on the body. The recipient may sit or lie and remains fully clothed. Reiki can also be used as a method of distant healing during which the practitioner works using visualization techniques. With both methods recipient consent is of paramount importance. R eiki energy is channelled for the 'greatest and highest good' of the recipient, and is understood to flow in response to the needs of the recipient. Recipients often report a feeling of deep relaxation during and following the therapy.

### Evidence base
Although there is some emerging evidence supporting the claims of both spiritual healing and therapeutic touch, the evidence for reiki to date is very small. The search for evidence did not find any studies carried out in supportive and palliative care.

Wardell & Engerretson's (2001) study examined the biological correlates of reiki healing. Twenty three healthy subjects received reiki lasting thirty minutes. The biological markers related to stress reduction response were measured pre and post reiki. These markers included breathing rate, pulse rate, blood pressure and salivary immunoglobulin levels. Significant biochemical and physiological changes in the direction of relaxation were noted. Although acknowledged as small, this study suggests that reiki would be a useful intervention for relaxation which warrants further study.

Despite lack of scientific evidence on the effects of reiki, anecdotal evidence suggests that reiki can assist in the care of patients in supportive and palliative care.

### Training
There are differing styles of reiki available today, which means that the number of levels of training will vary from one style to another. It is generally accepted that level 1 is mostly for personal use and for use in an informal way with friends and family. Practitioners of reiki in supportive and palliative care should be trained to practitioner level 2. There is also the master/teacher level which some approach as level 3, while others divide master level into master practitioner level 3, and master teacher level

4. At present, the standards of courses vary greatly. The UK Reiki Federation is currently laying the foundations for a core curriculum, and information can be found on their website: www.reikifed.co.uk. Other reiki organisations are in the process of being consulted on how best to carry the accreditation process forward.

Practitioners of reiki in supportive and palliative care should have transferable skills, relevant experience, or receive additional training in order to be able to decide on the suitability of reiki for use on vulnerable adults who are seriously or chronically ill, and take the necessary precautions. Refer to contraindications and precautions mentioned in 14.2.

## 14.4 Spiritual healing

### Brief description
Spiritual Healing is an ancient therapy which has been used throughout recorded history. Pythagoras (6 BC) considered healing to be the noblest of his pursuits and integrated it into his considerations of ethics: mind and soul. (Benor 2001) Spiritual healing, often referred to simply as healing, is a process that promotes better health, through the channelling of healing energies through the healer to the patient. (National Federation of Spiritual Healers 1998) Healing is said to quicken the body's natural healing processes on all levels. (Neate and Neate 2001) It is a supportive approach which may involve light touch or no touch at all, depending on the recipient's condition and wishes.

Healers view human life as four-dimensional, comprising body, emotions, mind and spirit. They are drawn to the work because of their interest in the spiritual dimension of life, and because they find they can transmit healing energy. Healers draw upon the finer energies of the universe, and they may or may not follow a particular religion. Many healers may embrace a spiritual understanding based on unconditional love. (Neate and Neate 2001)

Healing is becoming accepted as a valid and credible therapy, offered in some medical centres as a complement to conventional medical treatment (BMA 1993). Healers do not usually relate to the disease entities of conventional medicine, but aim to help the patient in more general terms, for example by increasing well-being. (Ernst 2001) The healer provides time for the patient to discuss problems, in order to gain some understanding of them; subsequently the patient may be asked to lie or sit down for treatment. (Ernst 2001)

### Evidence base
At the moment there is a paucity of clinical trials to support the efficacy of spiritual healing. Benor (2001) writes about the scientific validation of

healing, giving brief descriptions of 191 controlled studies across a broad range of conditions and organisms. Over 50% of the trials are said to result in a significant outcome in favour of healing. However, Benor himself points out the methodological flaws, and his interpretation of the evidence is unconventional. (Abbott 2002) Other authors reporting on the same trials conclude that the findings cannot be relied upon to draw firm conclusions about the efficacy or inefficacy of healing. (Abbot 2000)

Despite the lack of evidence, spiritual healing remains a popular therapy in supportive and palliative care. (Macmillan 2002)

### Training
Training for spiritual healers is currently provided by many professional organisations and usually takes about two years. This period involves attendance at formal training courses, supervised healing practice and documented records of ongoing personal development. During the training period healers are known as probationary healers, student healers or trainees. The development of standards of good practice, by UK Healers, along the lines of the national occupational standards for complementary therapies, is underway. Probationary, student or trainee healers are assessed by a panel prior to acceptance for registration with a regulatory body.

## 14.5 Therapeutic touch

### Brief description
Therapeutic touch emerged in the 1970s, introduced into mainstream nursing education by Dr. Dolores Krieger, then professor of nursing at New York University. Krieger had experienced the laying on of hands and was convinced that this was a natural potential inherent in everyone, which could be realised if the intention to help or heal was present. Therapeutic touch is without religious association, has been studied and researched within a healthcare framework, and has been introduced into nursing programmes in the USA at masters and doctorate levels. It has been taught at degree level in the UK for the last ten years.

Therapeutic touch has been considered as a contemporary interpretation of several ancient healing practices. Whilst honouring and respecting the influence of other traditions, it is within a framework which uses the insight of modern quantum physics that therapeutic touch is described. (Chopra 1989, Rogers 1983) It has also been described as an attempt to focus completely on the well-being of the patient in an act of unconditional love and compassion. (Quinn & Strelkkaukas 1993) This is not seen as a desire to cure or an attachment to a particular outcome.

Therapeutic touch is not regarded as involving channelling of energy or an energy exchange but as a mutual process, a healing meditation. It has been suggested that undergoing this process with a practitioner who is 'centred' (in a calm, alert and open state of consciousness with a clear sense of oneself and being connected to the holistic nature of healing, Sayre Adams & Wright 2001) brings about a change with the practitioner acting as a template to facilitate this change towards wholeness. (Quinn 1992)

During a treatment, the practitioner's hands are moved in a rhythmic, downward movement, a short distance away from the body of the client, starting at the head and working towards the feet. During this process the practitioner makes an assessment and may become aware of some imbalances in what is described (not without controversy) as the energy field. The practitioner then works towards 'clearing' these areas and promoting a sense of harmony and wholeness. Clients usually experience a deep relaxation response and anecdotal evidence suggests that they can become clearer about problems they are facing and feel less anxious generally.

### Evidence base
The following are studies relevant to palliative care and which provide evidence on the efficacy of therapeutic touch. A full overview and analysis can be found in the text by Sayre Adams & Wright (2001).

### a) Relaxation Response
Krieger et al's (1979) study demonstrated a deep relaxation response being present in clients receiving therapeutic touch. This was verified by ECG, EEG and electro–oculo graphic responses. Electro–myographic, hand temperature and galvanic skin responses were also recorded. Interestingly, the EEG of the practitioner demonstrated a predominant amount of fast synchronous beta activity, demonstrating intense concentration. Patients showed a high amount of alpha activity, which indicates a deep state of relaxation. This was a small study and has some flaws in its design. However, its findings are not without significance.

In Heidt's (1981) study ninety hospitalised cardiovascular patients were randomised into three groups. One group received therapeutic touch for five minutes, another group (control) received casual touch and the third had a nurse who talked to them for the five minutes test time. Pre and post test anxiety was assessed using the State-Trait[2] Anxiety Inventory (Spielberger 1983), a self-evaluation tool. The experimental group was found to have a statistically significant greater reduction in state

2 State anxiety can be described as stress /anxiety felt at the time, and trait anxiety as stress/anxiety felt 'normally'

anxiety scores than the other two groups. A criticism of this study is that the experimental group were aware that they were having therapeutic touch and therefore the placebo effect cannot be ruled out.

Quinn's (1982) sixty hospitalised patients with cardio- vascular conditions were randomly assigned to two groups. One group received a mimic treatment from three nurses with no knowledge of therapeutic touch, the other received therapeutic touch. Both treatments lasted for five minutes. Quinn's hypothesis that the therapeutic touch group would have a greater reduction in post test-trait anxiety scores (using the Spielberger State-Trait Anxiety Inventory 1983) was supported. This result also indicated that therapeutic touch involves an energy interaction, but the study does not attempt to draw conclusions as to defining its exact nature.

Quinn (1989 b) replicated the above study, with thirty-eight women and one hundred & fifteen men, all awaiting open heart surgery the following day, who were treated with either mimic therapeutic touch or therapeutic touch. The same assessment, using the State-Trait Anxiety Inventory, was used as previously. Blood pressure and heart rate were recorded pre and post test using separate analyses of co variance. Although no significant differences were recorded between the two groups, all post test measures did improve.

It must be noted that, where as in the 1982 study mimic therapeutic touch was given by nurses with no knowledge of therapeutic touch, in this study therapeutic touch and mimic therapeutic touch were given by therapeutic touch practitioners. Therefore it is possible that this influenced the small differential between groups. Similarly the shortness of length of the treatment has been questioned.

Olsen's (1992) study took place in the two months following hurricane Hugo in the United States. A convenience sample of twenty three volunteers, who had all experienced personal stress was used. A repeated session design was used with data collected before during and after each session. Physiological measurements such as blood pressure and skin temperature were included. The psychological variables were state anxiety and trait anxiety. These were tested by two visual analogue questionnaires. The findings showed that mean state anxiety scores decreased significantly after the therapeutic touch sessions, but that trait anxiety scores remained similar pre and post test. Physiological outcomes indicated a trend towards relaxation but these were not statistically significant.

b) Pain
Using a sample of sixty people, one group was treated with mimic therapeutic touch and the other with therapeutic touch. (Keller & Bzdek 1986) The

hypothesis was that the therapeutic touch group would experience greater relief from headache and that this would persist for four hours post treatment. The research design was rigorous and appropriate assessment tools were used. The hypothesis was supported, with statistically significant results.

This was a single, randomised control trial to determine the effect of therapeutic touch on osteoarthritis of the knee. (Gordon et al 1998). This was a small sample of twenty five, but significant differences were found in improvement in function and pain for those who received therapeutic touch.

In addition to supporting the hypothesis relating to pain, these studies also support the hypothesis that there is an energy interaction occurring during therapeutic touch.

c) Sleep
Using the Sleep Quality questionnaire as a measure, it was found that five out of six elderly subjects had a better quality of sleep during nights when therapeutic touch had been administered to them at bedtime. (Braun et al 1986)

d) Audit & evaluation of service
In Hallett's (1996) survey with oncology patients, following therapeutic touch:
- 75% said they were coping better (20% were coping the same)
- 70% reported feeling less anxious
- 47.5% felt happier
- 75% felt more peaceful and calm

Other responses included coping better with chemotherapy and radiotherapy (32.5%) 40% reported feeling more in control and 37.5% felt therapeutic touch had helped them to adjust to their diagnosis. A similar survey was conducted (Hallett 2000) and findings were very similar.

In summary, both research and anecdotal evidence indicate that therapeutic touch is helpful from a quality of life perspective and, for some, can be perceived as a deep and meaningful experience.

Training
Training in therapeutic touch is available at two levels. A two day introductory course introduces health care professionals to the main principles of therapeutic touch and is a pre-requisite to the full, advanced practitioner training. The course that leads to full, advanced practitioner status takes eight months and can be undertaken as an independent module or as a module within the degree for health care studies. Currently the only practitioner training course is in Lancaster, validated by St. Martin's College, University of Lancaster. Information on training can be obtained from the website of The Sacred Space Foundation, www.sacredspace.org.uk

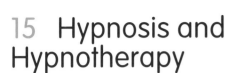

# 15 Hypnosis and Hypnotherapy

## 15.1 Brief description

Hypnosis has been described as a psychological state in which certain human capacities are heightened while others fade into the background. During hypnosis a person's critical faculty or logical mind is suspended or diminished, leading to an increase in the probability of the acceptance of therapeutic interventions. (Hawkins 1994, cited in Liossi and Mystakidou 1996) The term hypnosis denotes an interaction between one person, the hypnotist, and another person or people, the subject or subjects. (Heap et al 2001) In this interaction the hypnotist attempts to influence the subject's perceptions, feelings, thinking and behaviour by asking them to concentrate on ideas and images that may evoke the intended effects. There are numerous theories but no universally accepted mechanism to explain all the phenomena of hypnosis.

Trance is ". .a waking state of awareness in which a person's attention is detached from his or her immediate environment and is absorbed by inner experiences such as feelings, cognition and imagery". (Heap 1996) Suggestion is the purposeful use of the phenomenon of trance and is at the heart of hypnosis. (Zahourek 2001)

Trance or change in the state of mind is akin to intense or focused concentration or attention, a state which may be induced by techniques such as deep relaxation routines, visualisation, imagery, guided imagery, autogenic training, neurolinguistic programming and meditation, as well as other situations such as music festivals, religious ceremonies and sporting events. (Finlay and Jones 1996, Owens 2002)

In hypnosis the imagination, rather than the intellect, is active. (Taylor 2002) Hypnosis is a valuable tool which involves interaction between body and mind, using the mind to affect therapeutic change, and can be instrumental in engendering coping strategies, helping people to connect with their inner being and activate innate healing forces. (Spiegel and Moore 1997, Owens 2002)

In a consultation, the clinician, by the use of rapport building and communication skills, establishes the needs of the patient and endeavours to remove any doubts, fears and misconceptions they may have about hypnosis. Close empathic rapport is the first stage of the hypnotic process, and is generally followed by induction, following which the patient is guided into a state of deep relaxation. Within this state communication is retained, and specific suggestions geared to that person's presenting concerns are made. The benefits, and growth of the patient's autonomy, are reinforced by self hypnosis techniques and by post hypnotic suggestions, through which the patient goes through the hypnotic procedures on their own.

Whilst it is recognised that relaxation is a core skill for occupational therapists, and physiotherapists use some relaxation techniques, increasingly physicians, nurses and allied health professionals are using relaxation and visualisation and other forms of guided imagery, frequently within a group format, in the field of supportive and palliative care. (Walker 1992; Cayrou and Dolbeault 1997) Within this context, a question not infrequently raised by practitioners of hypnosis is 'are these conventional healthcare practitioners in fact using hypnosis?' It is advisable that practitioners who use hypnotic techniques, such as relaxation, visualisation and guided imagery within their field of work should have received formal instruction and training and be cognisant of the contraindications and precautions described later in this chapter.

## 15.2 Evidence

### As an adjunct to more conventional forms of psychotherapy

There is substantial evidence that hypnosis can be a valuable adjunct to more conventional forms of psychotherapy. The following are some examples.

Kirsch et al (1995) carried out a meta-analysis on 18 studies in which cognitive-behavioural therapy was compared with the same therapy supplemented by hypnosis. The results indicated that the addition of hypnosis substantially enhanced treatment outcome, so that the average client receiving cognitive-behavioural hypnotherapy showed greater improvement than at least 70% of clients receiving non-hypnotic treatment.

Similarly, Schoenberger (2000) writes of the growing body of research evaluating the use of hypnosis with cognitive-behavioural techniques in the treatment of psychological disorders. Overall, studies demonstrate a substantial benefit from the addition of hypnosis.

Lynn S J et al, (2000) summarised the evidence for the effectiveness of hypnosis as an empirically supported clinical intervention. Indications are, that as a whole, the clinical research to date generally substantiates the claim that hypnotic procedures can ameliorate some psychological and medical conditions.

Bejenke (2000) writes of the benefits of early intervention with cancer patients in a study based upon fifteen years of clinical practice. The use of hypnosis, including imagery and psychoneuroimmunological modalities, as a preparation for surgery, chemotherapy, radiation and bone marrow transplantation can reduce physical suffering and treatment side effects, and facilitate patient management.

Trijsburg et al (1992) reviews twenty-two studies on the effects of psychological treatment on cancer patients. Behavioural interventions and hypnosis were effective with respect to specific symptoms such as anxiety, pain, nausea, and vomiting.

Levitan (1992) describes a number of specific applications of hypnosis within cancer care. Hypnosis has unique advantages for patients, including improvement of self-esteem, involvement in self-care, return of locus of control, lack of unpleasant side effects and continued efficacy.

Stetter et al (2002) carried out a meta-analysis to evaluate the clinical effectiveness of autogenic training. Seventy-three controlled outcome studies were found (published 1952-99). Sixty studies (35 randomized controlled trials) qualified for inclusion in the meta-analysis.

### In the context of cancer management

Typically a person having cancer may encounter a series of 'pulses' of need for intervention as the disease and its treatment follow their course. Major concerns of the patient may be in relation to physical, psychological, emotional or spiritual distress. Interventions in the management of cancer, typically surgery, chemotherapy and radiotherapy, can be unpleasant, and will often become central to a patient's fears, anxieties and concerns, and may be addressed using hypnosis.

Certain concerns are not limited specifically to the cancer experience, but may be of a more general nature, for example panic attacks and needle phobia, and this will be evident in the references cited. This section attempts to identify the value of hypnosis in the management of some of the many crises occurring within the cancer journey. See Walker 1992.

### a) Emotional response to cancer

Spiegel (1990) states that patient resources for coping with breast cancer can be enhanced by attention to cognitive, affective, psychosomatic and social components of the illness. Systematic studies of such treatment interventions have shown favourable results, including significant reductions in mood disturbance and pain.

Walker et al (1999) examined the relationship between stress and response to chemotherapy.

They stated that the diagnosis and treatment of breast cancer are stressful, and stress may be associated with a poorer response to chemotherapy. There is a need, therefore, to develop and evaluate interventions that might enhance quality of life and, possibly, improve treatment response. The effects of relaxation combined with guided imagery (visualising host defences destroying tumour cells) on quality of life and response to primary chemotherapy, to date, have not been adequately evaluated.

Ninety-six women with newly diagnosed large or locally advanced breast cancer took part in a prospective, randomized controlled trial. As hypothesised, patients in the experimental group were more relaxed and easy going during the study, according to the Mood Rating Scale. (Anderson et al 2000) Quality of life was better in the experimental group, as assessed using the Global Self-assessment (Walker et al 1999) and Rotterdam Symptom Checklist. (De Haes et al 1990) The intervention also reduced emotional suppression, as measured by the Courtauld Emotional Control Scale (Watson and Greer 1983). The incidence of clinically significant mood disturbance was very low and the incidence in the two groups was similar. Finally, although the groups did not differ for clinical or pathological response to chemotherapy, imagery ratings were correlated with clinical response. These simple, inexpensive and beneficial interventions should be offered to patients wishing to improve quality of life during primary chemotherapy.

### b) Adjunctive to surgery

Montgomery et al, (2002) carried out a meta-analytical review of studies using hypnosis with surgical patients. The results indicated that patients in hypnosis treatment groups had better clinical outcomes than 89% of patients in control groups. These data strongly support the use of hypnosis with surgical patients.

### c) Chemotherapy related nausea and vomiting

Marchioro et al (2000) reported on 16 consecutive adult cancer patients affected by chemotherapy induced anticipatory nausea and vomiting who had received at least four treatment cycles. The experience highlights the potential value of hypnosis in the management of anticipatory nausea and vomiting.

Jacknow et al (1994) studied the effectiveness of hypnosis for decreasing antiemetic medication usage and treatment of chemotherapy related nausea and vomiting in children with cancer. Results suggest self-hypnosis is effective for decreasing antiemetic medication usage and for reducing anticipatory nausea during chemotherapy.

Burish T G et al (1983) report that some adverse side effects of cancer chemotherapy are attributed to the pharmacologic properties of the anti-neoplastic drugs, while others appear to be conditioned or learned. The literature suggests that behavioural relaxation techniques can significantly alleviate some conditioned side effects of chemotherapy including nausea, vomiting and negative emotions such as anxiety and depression. These behavioural procedures are generally inexpensive, easily learned, and have few if any negative side effects.

Walker et al (1988) describe a promising psychological treatment for ameliorating the side effects of cytotoxic chemotherapy used in cancer treatment. It is brief, does not require the therapist to be present immediately before or during chemotherapy, and does not need to be carried out in the same clinical area as the chemotherapy. Fourteen patients, all of whom had severe side effects, took part in an open clinical trial. All patients, including two who had previously refused further chemotherapy, completed their prescribed course of chemotherapy. In a number of patients, impressive improvements were observed in conditioned nausea and vomiting, pharmacological nausea and vomiting and other symptoms.

In a study by Zeltzer L et al (1984) fifty-one children 6-17 years of age rated the severity of nausea, vomiting, and the extent to which chemotherapy bothered them during each course of chemotherapy. The data indicate that chemotherapy related nausea and emesis in children can be reduced with behavioural intervention and that reductions are maintained after intervention has been discontinued. See also Walker et al 1990.

### d) Scanning and radiotherapy procedures
Friday et al (1990) reported on the use of hypnosis as an intervention in MRI procedure. Medical hypnosis has been an effective intervention in ten patients, permitting completion of their diagnostic procedure. See also Steggles 1999.

### e) Pain
Syrjala K L et al (1995) compared oral mucositis pain levels in four groups of cancer patients receiving bone marrow transplants. From results obtained the conclusion is that relaxation and imagery training reduces cancer treatment related pain. The results from other studies also indicate that pain in cancer care responds well to hypnosis.

Spiegel & Bloom (1983) studied the pain and mood disturbance of 54 women with metastatic carcinoma of the breast over the course of one year. Those who were offered the self-hypnosis training as well as group therapy fared best in controlling the pain sensation. Pain frequency and duration were not affected.

### f) In advanced cancer
Liossi & White (2001) carried out research to evaluate the efficacy of clinical hypnosis in the enhancement of quality of life of patients with far-advanced cancer. The study concluded that hypnosis is effective in the enhancement of quality of life in terminally ill cancer patients.

### g) Immune response
Lynn et al (2000) report the results of an 18-month study of immune system and psychological changes in stage 1 breast cancer patients provided with relaxation, guided imagery, and biofeedback training. The results show that behavioural interventions can be correlated with immune system measures, thereby replicating the results of an earlier pilot study.

Spiegel & Moore (1997) report on a 10-year follow-up of a randomized trial involving 86 women with cancer which showed that a year of weekly supportive, expressive group therapy significantly increased survival duration and time from recurrence to death.

Johnson et al (1996) carried out a study with the aims of evaluating the psychological and immunological effects of 3 weeks' relaxation practice; investigating the effects of relaxation training and hypnosis on the modulation of the immune response to an experimental stressor; and relating changes to hypnotic susceptibility. A conclusion was that hypnotisability may be an important moderator of the psychoneuroimmunological response to relaxation training and exposure to acute stress.

Walker (1998) states that in recent years it has become increasingly clear that the diagnosis and treatment of cancer are stressful experiences. Not surprisingly, therefore, high levels of psychiatric morbidity and psychological distress have been reported. (Derogatis et al 1983) There is now evidence, however, from prospective, randomized controlled trials that psychological interventions can enhance the quality of life of patients with cancer (see Meyer and Mark, 1995 for a meta-analysis). In addition, psychological interventions, including hypnosis, can modulate the immune response in a way that might be relevant to the progression of malignant disease. (Walker and Eremin, 1995) See also Walker (1992)

In summary, a large body of evidence exists for the use of clinical hypnosis and hypnosis may be useful in supportive and palliative care for in the following ways:

- **To enhance the immune response** (Walker 1992, Walker & Eremin 1995, Johnson et al 1996, Spiegel & Moore 1997, Walker 1988, Lynn et al 2000)

- **As an adjunct to more conventional forms of psychotherapy** (Levitan 1992, Kirsch et al 1995, Schoenberger 2000, Lynn et al 2000, Bejenke 2000)
- **To enhance coping ability** (Walker 1992, Levitan 1992, Walker 1999)
- **To enhance recovery from surgery** (Montgomery et al 2002)
- **To reduce chemotherapy-related nausea and vomiting** (Burish et al 1983, Walker 1988, Walker 1992, Jacknow et al 1994, Marchioro et al 2000)
- **To increase tolerance of scanning and radiotherapy procedures** (Friday et al 1990, Walker 1992, Steggles 1999)
- **To reduce pain** (Syrjala et al 1995, Spiegel & Bloom 1983, Trijsburg et al 1992)
- **In mood disturbance and emotional and psychological distress** (Spiegel 1990, Walker 1992, Lynn et al 2000)
- **To enhance quality of life** (Levitan 1992, Walker 1999)
- **To reduce anxiety and depression** (Trijsburg et al 1992, Burish et al 1983)

## 15.3 Use of hypnosis in supportive and palliative care

### Contraindications
- Psychiatric status: where any psychiatric condition exists which may lead to unpredictable behaviour and responses, hypnosis is contraindicated.
- Emotional status: depression is often a concomitant of cancer. Effective treatment of depression in cancer patients results in better patient adjustment, reduced symptoms, reduced cost of care, and may influence disease course (Spiegel 1996). When using hypnosis, the lack of clinical expertise specifically in working with the depressed person may only serve to compound their problem.

### Precautions
- **Be aware** of inexpert use. Clinicians should not work outside their own areas of training and competence. Stanley et al (1998) state that increasingly there is developing a conviction that the hypnotic state or process itself poses no inherent dangers for patients but that its inexpert use may. The solution to prevent potential patient harm is to ensure that all clinicians of whatever discipline have adequate and appropriate clinical training prior to being allowed to practise.

"With….real authorities, agreement is almost unanimous that dangers (of hypnosis) are minimal and can be avoided. In some instances there have been bad results, but they have come because of personality difficulties of the hypnotist, authoritative, coercive use of hypnosis, or lack of

knowledge. Patients will protect themselves from harm when the therapist shows respect for their ability to do so" (Cheek & Le Cron 1968).

- **Explain** to the patient the likely process of the hypnotic intervention, to remove any doubts and fears, and to obtain the approval and consent of the patient.

- **Be aware** of the legal implications of working with a patient who is in a state of hyper-suggestibility, and who, generally, will have their eyes closed.

- **Be aware** that abreaction, a (possibly powerful) emotional response to recalled images and feelings, may be triggered in hypnosis. This is particularly likely where the patient is already under considerable emotional pressure. The clinician should be trained and competent in using skills to protect and work with the patient, and to re-orientate the patient following an abreaction.

- **Remove** any suggestion other than those intended to be post hypnotic, before 'alerting' a patient. For example, if anaesthesia had been produced it is important to terminate it. (Cheek & Le Cron 1968)

- **Ensure** post hypnotic suggestions are time and situation specific.

- **Ensure** the patient is brought out of the hypnotic state gradually.

- **Ensure** the patient is fully awake and alert before concluding the session.

## 15.4 Regulation and training

Chapter 5 should be referred to for the current position on regulation and training of complementary therapy professions. The regulation of hypnotherapists under a single regulatory body is at an early stage and a working group that is inclusive of all the different organisations and facilitated by an independent chair, has not been agreed. Further information can be obtained from The Prince of Wales's Foundation for Integrated Health www.fihealth.org.uk

### Regulation
British Society of Medical and Dental Hypnosis and its branches, and The British Society of Experimental and Clinical Hypnosis are the two professional organisations in the UK whose members practise hypnosis integrated with the professional's primary conventional health care role. Members are answerable to, and follow the codes of ethics, conduct, etc of their relevant regulatory body, for instance the General Medical Council, or Nursing and Midwifery Council.

Members of the British Society of Medical and Dental Hypnosis are encouraged to work towards accreditation, and accredited members are listed on the Society referral register. Details can be obtained from the national office.

Hypnotherapists who are also psychotherapists are registered with the United Kingdom Council for Psychotherapists. Information can be obtained by writing to the United Kingdom Council for Psychotherapists email: UKCP@psychotherapy.org.uk

There are a large number of professional organisations that register hypnotherapists who have trained with organisations other than the British Society of Medical and Dental Hypnosis. The UK Confederation of Hypnotherapy Organisations is the umbrella body for a number of organisations, see www.ukcho.org. There are also hypnotherapy organisations who are not members of UKCHO.

Training

The British Society of Medical and Dental Hypnosis is a national and federal organisation which offers training in hypnosis to professionals with a conventional health care qualification who are employed in a substantive post with the NHS. Training is at basic, intermediate and advanced levels and members are encouraged to pursue training towards accreditation by the British Society of Medical and Dental Hypnosis. The core curriculum is set at national level and training is organised at branch level. In order to maintain consistent standards, a selection of branch level courses are attended annually by observers from other branches. Details of training courses can be obtained from the British Society of Medical and Dental Hypnosis national office. Tel/fax: 07000 560309, email: nat.office@bsmdh.org Website: www.bsmdh.org

The British Society of Medical and Dental Hypnosis view hypnosis as an additional skill or tool for professionals with a conventional health care qualification, to be used alongside their primary role as a doctor, dentist or nurse and within the expertise of their primary qualification. From the perspective of the British Society of Medical and Dental Hypnosis, the ethics and clinical responsibility that come with working with a person in a hypnotised state are such that those practising hypnosis should already have a primary professional relationship with the patient, be able to accept clinical responsibility for their actions, and have indemnity cover. Some members of the Society go for further training in psychotherapy or hypnotherapy.

The British Society of Experimental and Clinical Hypnosis works closely with the British Society of Medical and Dental Hypnosis and offers some courses, but does not accredit practitioners.

Although open to other professionals, membership comprises mainly psychologists who may or may not be trained in hypnosis.

The Department of Hypnosis at University College London offers training to appropriate conventional health care practitioners to diploma and MSc level in clinical and applied hypnosis. Contact Dr. David Oakley at ucjtcpl@ucl.ac.uk. Graduates are eligible for membership of The British Society of Medical and Dental Hypnosis or The British Society of Experimental and Clinical Hypnosis, and also to apply for accreditation. Glasgow Caledonian University has introduced a diploma course this year.

Apart from the British Society of Medical and Dental Hypnosis, hypnotherapists also train at a large number of other establishments and professional organisations. The level of training varies, and there is at present no agreed standard or core curriculum. The second edition of national occupational standards for hypnotherapy is currently being developed. These are the minimum agreed standards to which practitioners should be able to work.

# 16 Acupuncture

## 16.1 Brief description

Acupuncture is a word derived from the Latin *acus*, needle and *pungere*, to pierce. It is a therapeutic technique that involves the insertion of fine needles into the skin and underlying tissues at specific points, for therapeutic or preventative purposes. (Ernst 2001) The origins of acupuncture go back at least 2,000 years in China (Ma 1992). Anthropologists and medical historians have described many ways in which sensory modulation has been used for therapeutic purposes over the years in different cultures (Melzack 1994). Indeed, Ötzi, the European Ice Man, discovered in the Alps in 1991 and dated 5,200 years old, had numerous tattoos on his body over areas which corresponded to areas of arthritis on imaging. (Dorfer 1999) The locations and asymmetry of the tattoos on the body suggests that they were not ornamental and many were at sites commonly used for acupuncture treatment, so it was concluded that they represented a therapeutic technique.

Traditional acupuncture is used to treat a wide variety of disorders. For many traditional acupuncturists, acupuncture is practised as part of Traditional Chinese Medicine. In Traditional Chinese Medicine a fundamental concept is qi (pronounced chee), which is usually translated as 'energy'. (Vickers and Zollmann 1999; Ernst 2001) The roots of the concept qi, and many of the most important traditional acupuncture concepts, are at the very heart of Chinese culture. Qi is associated with the image of a warm hearth, a full stomach, and a sense of well-being. (Birch and Felt 1999) A person's qi, or energy, is present at birth and circulates throughout the body maintaining its physiological functions. When qi is fully dissipated death occurs. The major pathways for its circulation are the meridians or channels that form a continuous network throughout the body. Another basic concept of health is the balancing of two opposites, yin and yang. By careful observation of the symptoms of someone who is ill, a practitioner can determine the nature of the disturbances in the flow of energy, and of the disharmony to the normal balance of yin and yang.

Practitioners who solely use the traditional, energetic concept of acupuncture will insert needles at acupuncture points for which credibility has been established empirically. The aim of this approach is described in terms of correcting the body's energy flow and restoration of balance. Traditional acupuncturists base their diagnosis on a careful discussion with the patient, which may take into account more than obvious signs and symptoms. In their overall diagnosis, they often incorporate a sophisticated pulse and tongue diagnosis in order to identify the underlying patterns of disharmony which will guide treatment. (Lu and Needham 1980; Kaptchuk 2000) Acupressure uses similar principles but without needles; it can be administered with local finger pressure or pressure bands.

Many western medical acupuncturists undertake initial extensive training in traditional acupuncture techniques. However neurophysiological and neuropharmacological advances in the study of acupuncture have caused them to challenge the credibility of the traditional energetic diagnostic approach. Recent neuropharmacological and neurophysiological advances have given acupuncture an additional scientific basis and far more clinical acceptability for sceptical opponents of the subject. For example, acupuncture's actions are blocked by pre-treatment with injection of local anaesthetic. (Chiang, et al, 1973; Research Group of Acupuncture Anaesthesia, 1973; Dundee and Ghaly, 1991) It releases b-endorphins (Sjolund et al, 1977; Clement-Jones et al, 1980), met-enkephalin and dynorphins, which work on MOR, DOR and KOR (mu, delta, and kappa) opioid receptors. (Han and Terenius 1982; Han et al, 1991) Oxytocin, which is anxiolytic and analgesic, is released. (Uvnas-Moberg et al, 1993) This in turn releases serotonin which has both analgesic and mood enhancing properties (Han and Terenius, 1982). It has widespread autonomic effects (Ernst and Lee, 1985; Lundeberg 1999) and releases endogenous steroids. (Roth et al, 1997) Acupuncture is thought to up-regulate endogenous opioid gene production (Guo et al, 1996) which explains why top-ups are required, in part to maintain the gene expression in a 'switched on' mode. (Zieglgänsberger 2002, personal communication)

Many theories have been put forward regarding the anatomical or physiological basis of acupuncture points and meridians. For example, functional magnetic resonance imaging (fMRI) has been used to detect activity in the visual and auditory lobes of the brain during needling of distal acupuncture points on the leg and foot, the locations being based on traditional acupuncture practice for the treatment of eye and ear dysfunctions. (Cho et al 1998, Cho et al 1999)

Many neurophysiological mechanisms are described in further detail by Bowsher (1998), Pomeranz (2001), White (1999), Lundeberg (1999), and Filshie and Thompson (in press). There is a 71% overlap between acupuncture and trigger points. (Melzack, Stillwell and Fox, 1977) Trigger point acupuncture is particularly effective for myofascial musculoskeletal pain (Baldry, 2001). The meridian pathways frequently coincide with the referral pattern of trigger points. (Filshie and Cummings, 1999) The diagnostic reliability of the pulse diagnosis has been questioned. (Vincent, 1992)

OK

Within the broad rubric of traditional acupuncture, there is considerable diversity in styles, for example, Chinese, Korean, Vietnamese and Japanese acupuncture, plus Chinese and French auriculoacupuncture or ear acupuncture. Many western medical acupuncturists often take a more pragmatic approach to treatment and use an eclectic mix of treatments, traditional and western medical approaches and many use microsystem acupuncture, for example ear acupuncture or auriculotherapy. Some have even simplified the treatment approach further, leaving the complex energetic approach to its historical context only. (Mann, 2000; Campbell, 2001; Baldry, 2001)

Acupuncture is currently performed in over 84% of pain clinics (Woollam and Jackson, 1998; CSAG, 2000). Twenty-one per cent of GP practices offer access to acupuncture. (Thomas 2001) Western medical acupuncture treatment is not restricted to pain treatment alone and is used for treatment of multiple problems including respiratory problems, gastro-intestinal symptoms, cardiac, neurological and gynaecological conditions. (Filshie and White, 1998) Western medical acupuncturists use a mixture of segmental points appropriate to the disordered segment, for example T1 and T2 when the intercostobrachial nerve is damaged in axillary dissection, trigger points, tender points, plus selected 'strong' traditional points which have been commonly used, many of which, for example LI4, are known to increase the pain threshold. (Brockhaus and Elger, 1990)

Western medical acupuncture is used following an orthodox diagnosis based on conventional history taking, examination and special investigations (Filshie and Thompson, in press). Traditional acupuncturists are trained in basic sciences and have some degree of training in conventional medicine to a level which enables them to recognise symptoms of a more serious nature or red flags. Where appropriate, they ensure that patients are referred to their GP or oncologist for further investigations. This is important as an energetic diagnosis alone is potentially dangerous in certain circumstances. (Filshie, 2001) As a result of this, specific training courses have been developed in the UK for palliative care physicians and other medical practitioners who wish to treat palliative care patients as have acupuncture courses to familiarise other doctors and acupuncture practitioners who work with cancer patients (see 16.4).

In palliative care, acupuncture is used alongside conventional medical treatment and has an increasing supportive role for pain and symptom management. (Filshie; 2001; Wong et al; 2001) Some practitioners advocate its use to enhance psycho-spiritual well-being. (Aung, 1994; Wong et al, 2001) Filshie and Thompson (2000) are more

circumspect, though they acknowledge that psychoneuroimmunomodulation can go part way to explain how acupuncture works on the body and the mind.

## 16.2 Evidence base

Significant positive evidence is now available based on systematic reviews and meta-analyses for the use of acupuncture for the control of nausea and vomiting (Vickers, 1996), postoperative nausea and vomiting (Lee and Done, 1999), experimental pain (White, 1999), dental pain (Ernst and Pitler, 1998), headache (Melchart, 1999) and fibromyalgia (Berman, 1999). Acupuncture treatment for back pain is somewhat more controversial with a positive review (Ernst and White, 1998), a negative review (Smith, 2000) and a rather neutral review (Van Tulder, 2000). Cummings (2000) has critically appraised these anomalies. Inconclusive evidence exists for stroke, asthma and neck pain and negative evidence for weight loss and smoking cessation (Ernst, 1999), though the results for this are comparable to the success of nicotine patches.

Based partly on Vickers' (1996) data on acupuncture for nausea and vomiting, the National Institutes of Health Consensus Statement on Acupuncture (NIH, 1997) recommended acceptance of acupuncture as a useful clinical modality of treatment.

Acupuncture has been used to treat acute postoperative pain in cancer patients and also chronic or intractable pain associated with the cancer or its various treatments, for example surgery and radiotherapy. It is also used for non-pain symptoms such as nausea and vomiting, dyspnoea, xerostomia and many other troublesome problems in palliative care.

The results of clinical trials of acupuncture for pain unrelated to cancer have often been conflicting, with inconclusive results based on heterogeneous data and greatly flawed methodology (Patel, 1989; Ter Riet, 1990). This is hardly surprising, as trial methodology for acupuncture studies is particularly complex (White, 2002). Though randomisation is possible, suitable 'blinding' of patients is problematic, as is the provision of a credible needleless placebo (White, 2001). However, depending on the research questions asked, it is possible to use an alternative non-acupuncture group for comparison. A more recent pain review by Ezzo et al (2000) was similarly inconclusive but showed some superiority of acupuncture treatment compared with untreated patients, and demonstrated a greater effect for invasive compared to non-invasive controls.

### Acute postoperative pain and symptom control

Acupuncture reduced per and post operative analgesic requirements in a randomised controlled trial of 250 patients undergoing major abdominal surgery for cancer (Poulain, 1997). Intradermal needles sited pre-operatively and remaining post operatively reduced post operative analgesic requirements in a study involving 191 patients having upper and lower gastrointestinal surgery. (Kotani et al, 2001) It also caused less pain and increased mobility in the post operative period for patients undergoing axillary dissection for breast cancer. (He et al, 1999) Acupuncture as an alternative to anaesthesia is risky, but as an adjunct can be very efficacious in reducing per and postoperative analgesic requirements.

### Chronic cancer and cancer treatment related pain

Acupuncture has been used quite extensively for control of chronic and treatment-related cancer pain. However, the majority of work relies on observational reports, audits and case series to date. It is notoriously difficult to recruit patients to clinical trials in palliative care (Faithful, 1996) and acupuncture is no exception. There is a high attrition rate for conventional studies (Kirkham, 1997), let alone studies in complementary medicine.

In summaries of two extensive audits (Filshie and Redman, 1985; Filshie, 1990), acupuncture was found to improve pain control and reduce analgesic requirements in patients who had failed to respond to conventional treatment, though top-ups were likely to be more frequent than with non-cancer patients. An increase in mobility often accompanied pain reduction.

Patients with cancer treatment related pains such as post-surgical syndromes or post-irradiation like pain respond better than patients with extensive disease. The more advanced the disease, the shorter the response to treatment. Any tolerance to treatment was often an indication for tumour recurrence and hence a warning to check on the cancer status of the patients. Leng (1999) showed similar results in a hospice-based audit. Pain control in abdominal cancer was also achieved for at least one month in a case series of patients with mild or moderate pain and 72% with severe pain. (Xu, Liu and Li, 1995) Wen (1977) gave several electroacupuncture treatments per day and then steadily reduced the number of treatments per day on patients who responded with uncontrolled pain. Percutaneous electrical nerve stimulation (PENS) is reported as a novel treatment but appears to be electroacupuncture with a new name. One report showed pain, secondary to bony metastases, to be improved in two out of three patients (Ahmed, 1998).

Aung (1994) combined acupuncture with Qi Gong and breathing exercises and meditation in his case series. A recent audit by Johnstone et al (2002) showed success for a range of symptoms including pain: 86% of patients considered it 'very important' to continue to provide an acupuncture service. An audit on patients with breast cancer related pain showed an improvement of depression scores in addition to improvement in pain, distress and interference with lifestyle. (Filshie et al, 1997) Maintenance of relief is often problematic in cancer patients and two studies showed the short-term improvement in pain control using semipermanent indwelling needles in the ear, auriculoacupuncture. The former included five patients with motor neurone disease. (Dillon and Lucas, 1999; Alimi, 2000)

### Nausea and vomiting

Numerous randomised controlled trials (RCTs) have been performed using mostly the traditional point PC6 with a variety of stimuli to reduce chemotherapy induced nausea and vomiting. The impact of uncontrolled nausea and vomiting may be significant and may even lead to patients abandoning chemotherapy due to the negative impact on quality of life. Prevention is more successful than treatment once it develops. Acupuncture, electroacupuncture, acupressure or transcutaneous electrical nerve stimulation (TENS) were all compared with a control treatment. Seven out of eight studies were positive (Dundee et al, 1987; Stannard, 1989; McMillan et al, 1991; Price et al, 1991; Dibble et al, 2000; Shen et al, 2000; Roscoe et al, 2002). Roscoe et al (2002), the negative study, used electrical stimulation at PC6 but did not stipulate the exact electrical parameters used and may have been different from those by the late John Dundee and Christine McMillan (1991) found to give optimal effect.

Andrew Vickers (1996) performed the first systematic review on acupuncture for nausea and vomiting and reviewed acupuncture for nausea and vomiting associated with surgery, cancer chemotherapy and morning sickness. The review concluded that, although the studies were not methodologically perfect, PC6 acupuncture seems to be an effective antiemetic technique, though somewhat less effective in some of the trials reviewed when administered under anaesthesia.

Numerous other subsequent reviews have come to similar conclusions. (Mayer, 2000; Jacobson, Workman and Kronenberg, 2000; Pan, 2000; Wong, Sagar and Sagar, 2001) However, a preliminary analysis of the Cochrane review (Richardson et al, 2001) examining the effectiveness of acupuncture for chemotherapy induced nausea and vomiting found that the stimulation of PC6 acupoint reduced vomiting during chemotherapy, but the effect appears to be short-term only. The challenge remains to compare adequately powered random controlled trials with newer antiemetics such as the 5HT-3 antagonist ondansetron.

Nausea and vomiting in advanced terminal care is considerably more complex and may be due to one or many of the following causes: gastrointestinal problems including intestinal obstruction; drugs, for example strong opioids like morphine; metabolic causes including hypercalcaemia and renal failure; brain metastases; or dehydration. The cause of the nausea and vomiting needs identifying by orthodox medical diagnosis and clinical tests as appropriate and acupuncture may or may not be indicated. If acupuncture is found to be of potential value, having excluded serious causes, points with known physiological effects such as ST36 (Tougas et al, 1992) or CV12 or ST25 may need to be added if reversible gastrointestinal dysfunction is contributing to the nausea and vomiting.

## Shortness of breath

In a single-blind random controlled trial on 24 patients with chronic obstructive pulmonary disease (COPD) and disabling shortness of breath, patients had significant benefit in subjective breathlessness with the use of traditional acupuncture compared with sham, and had an increased 6-minute walking distance, though objective measures were unchanged (Jobst et al, 1986). In a further single-blind, randomised crossover study, 31 patients with severe **COPD** were taught to practice acupressure daily for 6 weeks, then sham acupressure for a further 6 weeks. Dyspnoea, as measured by a visual analogue scale, was significantly less with real acupressure (Maa et al 1997). Ernst's (2001) review concluded that, despite the paucity of trials, there is data to support the use of acupuncture and acupressure to relieve dyspnoea towards the end of life for patients with severe chronic obstructive pulmonary disease.

A pilot study of 20 patients (Filshie et al, 1996) with cancer related breathlessness at rest, who were treated with acupuncture at points on the upper 5 cms of the sternum and LI 4 for 10 minutes, found that 70% of patients reported a marked symptomatic improvement; there were significant improvement in visual analogue scores of breathlessness, relaxation and anxiety that peaked at 90 minutes and lasted up to 6 hours. Respiratory rate also significantly decreased. Semipermanent indwelling needles were used to prolong the effect. These can remain in place covered by a clear plastic dressing for up to four weeks at a time to give patients immediate control by massaging them in the event of a panic attack or prior to any, even trivial exercise. (Filshie and Thompson, in press)

## Xerostomia

Acupuncture has been shown to improve the unpleasant symptoms of xerostomia due to a variety of causes. Blom and Dawidson's team have performed many studies, including an RCT on 38 patients with xerostomia following radiotherapy that showed both classical and superficial acupuncture to increase salivary flow (Blom et al, 1996). In another study, 50% of patients with xerostomia, who were refractory to pilocarpine, were also helped. (Johnstone et al, 2001) Lundeberg has described many of the physiological principles by which it is known to work (Lundeberg, 1999). Acupuncture has also helped patients in late stage palliative care for xerostomia dysphagia and articulation problems. (Rydholm and Strang, 1999)

## Cancer-related hot flushes

Acupuncture has been found to be helpful for hot flushes due to the natural climacteric. (Wyon et al, 1994). Acupuncture can reduce the hot flushes associated with hormone manipulation in breast cancer care following tamoxifen (Cumins et al, 2000). Semipermanent needles inserted in SP6 can help to maintain the effect in patients who fail to respond to a short course of weekly treatments (Towlerton et al, 1999). Acupuncture has also helped patients with prostate cancer undergoing hormone treatment. (Hammar, 1999)

## Anxiety and depression

The use of indwelling anxiety, sickness and dyspnoea (ASAD) points on the upper 5 cms of the sternum has been found to be useful for anxiety as well as dyspnoea and in some cases nausea, though not formally tested. (Filshie and Thompson, in press) Patients can stimulate the semipermanent needles covered by a clear plastic dressing by gently massaging over the needles when they are particularly anxious, and this can have a rapid calming effect in responders. Though acupuncture has been found to be equally as helpful as tricyclic drugs, (Ernst et al, 1998) there are also many newer drugs which are reliable for the treatment of depression in this group of patients. Patients attending for physical complaints have often experienced marked changes to their emotional and mental states (Gould & MacPherson 2001), supporting claims of a lift in mood occurring concurrently with a course of acupuncture treatment.

## People with HIV/AIDS

Forty-eight per cent of 1016 patients with AIDS used acupuncture to treat their symptoms (Green et al, 1999). Though acupuncture has been found helpful for sleep disturbance (Philips and Skelton 2001), a large random controlled trial comparing acupuncture with amitriptyline and placebo failed to show any benefit of acupuncture over the other treatments for pain of peripheral neuropathy. (Shlay et al, 1998)

## Miscellaneous

Patients with cancer often present with non-cancer related symptoms. A prospective and descriptive study with 291 acupuncture patients showed a reduction in symptoms, such as musculoskeletal, respiratory, psychological, and neurological, in the majority of patients. (Chapman, Norton and Paterson 2001) The outcome measure used was the Measure Yourself Medical Outcome Profile questionnaire.

Acupuncture has been found to be helpful for a variety of vascular problems including angina and ischaemic skin flaps, (Lundeberg, 1999) and even radionecrotic ulcers have been healed, which classically do not heal (Filshie, 1988). Acupuncture has also helped intractable hiccup, (Yan 1988) dysphagia due to oesophageal obstruction, (Feng, 1984) radiation rectitis (Zhang, 1987) and uraemic pruritis (Duo, 1987).

In summary, current evidence supports the use of acupuncture and acupressure in palliative care for chemotherapy induced and post operative nausea and vomiting with high level evidence emerging for acute pain and xerostomia. Despite the limited scientific evidence, there is data to support the use of acupuncture for other symptoms, and it may be useful in supportive and palliative care for the following conditions.

- **Chemotherapy-induced and post-operative nausea and vomiting** (Dundee et al, 1987; Stannard, 1989; McMillan et al, 1991; Price et al, 1991; Dibble et al, 200; Shen et al, 2000; Aglietti, 1990; Roscoe et al, 2002. Reviews: Vickers, 1996, Richardson et al, 2001. Postoperative nausea and vomiting: Lee and Done, 1999)
- **Pain relief** (Acute pain: Poulain, 1997; Kotani, 2001; He et al, 1999. Chronic pain: Wen, 1977; Filshie and Redman, 1985; Filshie, 1990; Aung, 1994; Thompson and Filshie, in press; Xu, Liu and Li, 1995; Filshie et al 1997; Dillon and Lucas, 1999; Leng, 1999; Filshie, 2000; Johnstone et al, 2002; Alimi et al, 2000)
- **Non-cancer related pain: musculoskeletal** (Baldry, 2001); **dental pain** (Ernst & Pittler 1998); **headache** (Melchart, Linde & Fisher 1999); **experimental pain** (White, 1999) **fibromyalgia** (Berman, 1999)
- **Breathlessness, including severe COPD and use of indwelling semi-permanent needles** (Jobst et al 1986; Filshie et al 1996; Maa et al 1997; Ernst 2001; Filshie and Thompson, in press)
- **Xerostomia (dry mouth)** (Blom et al 1992; Blom et al 1993; Talal et al 1992; Blom, 1996; Blom & Lundberg 2000; Johnstone et al 2002)
- **Radiation induced rectitis** (Zhang 1987)
- **Hiccups** (Yan, 1988)
- **Hot flushes, including semi-permanent indwelling needles** (Wyon, 1998; Towlerton, Filshie et al 1999; Hammar, 1999; Cumins, 2000; Johnstone et al 2002)
- **Angina** (Richter et al 1991; Ballegaard et al, 1995)
- **AIDS** (Philips and Skelton, 2001)

## 16.3 Use of acupuncture in supportive and palliative care

### Contraindications
- **Avoid** any area of actual or potential spinal instability due to cancer. It potentially increases the risk of cord compression or transection
- **Avoid** inserting needles directly over the tumour itself or nodules or related sites, such as ascites
- **Do not** use acupuncture in severely disordered clotting function
- **Avoid** indwelling needles with patients at risk of bacteraemia, for instance in valvular heart disease and immunocompromised patients with neutropenia
- **Avoid** needling a lymphoedematous limb
- **Avoid** needling directly above a prosthesis
- **Avoid** needling over any intracranial deficits following neurosurgery

### Precautions
- **Only use** sterile, single-use disposable needles
- **Take particular care** when needling over the ribcage and the domes of the pleura, especially in cachectic patients and the hyperinflated chests of patients with chronic obstructive pulmonary disease
- **To reduce the risk** of pneumothorax, paravertebral needling or needles to the top of the sternum are useful alternatives
- **Avoid** the arm on the side of mastectomy and/or axillary lymph gland dissection
- **Be aware** that if tolerance occurs, it may represent progressive disease and full investigation of tumour status may be required
- **Caution** with indwelling semipermanent needles in any strong reactor to acupuncture
- **Be aware** that patients may be undergoing chemotherapy, radiotherapy or hormonal treatments (refer to Chapter 10, Clinical Issues)
- **Be aware** that patients may be particularly fatigued and are living with a chronic/life-threatening illness (see Section 10, Clinical Issues)
- **Be aware** that acupuncture can mask both cancer and disease progression
- **Use** acupuncture with caution where the patient's behaviour is unpredictable

Additionally, any advice about offering acupuncture as an alternative to conventional treatment or over optimism about the potential for helping any patient is clearly inappropriate. In cases where patients are angry or in denial about their illness, practitioners will need to be especially sensitive and skilful. (Filshie, 2001)

### Safety
In the hands of appropriately qualified health professionals, acupuncture seems safe (Vincent,

2001). Professional bodies that register practitioners of acupuncture issue clinical standards and guidelines for safe practice. In addition, practitioners should be familiar with recent publications on safety issues (Filshie 2001; MacPherson et al 2001; White et al 2001; Peuker and Gronemeyer 2001, Walsh 2001, Hoffman 2001). In particular, the article by Filshie (2001), which outlines specific problems of acupuncture in cancer patients, is recommended reading. For ease of reference, these articles can be downloaded from the website of the British Medical Acupuncture Society www.medical-acupuncture.co.uk

**a) Serious adverse effects**
Serious adverse effects are well recognised but rare, and Peuker and Gronemeyer (2001) reviewed rare but serious complications of acupuncture including:
- Delayed or missed diagnosis of the condition treated. Acupuncture can mask both cancer and disease progression (Filshie 2001)
- Trauma to tissues and organs
- Pneumothorax. This is a particular hazard in patients with thin chest walls, and cachectic patients will therefore be at particular risk.
- Bacterial and viral infections, hepatitis B, C and HIV. (Walsh 2001) The introduction of infection through bacteraemia, septicaemia in immunocompromised patients, and endocarditis in patients with heart valve lesions. Using single use disposable needles has dramatically reduced the risk of spread of hepatitis B and C infections.

**b) Mild reactions**
Relatively mild reactions to treatment are common. Two recent large prospective surveys of adverse events associated with acupuncture, involving a total of 66,000 patients, showed a low incidence of significant minor adverse events, 13 per 10,000 or less, though the number of cancer patients treated in the samples was unspecified. (White et al, 2001; MacPherson et al, 2001)
- Bleeding (3%) and pain at the site of needling (1%) are common local reactions. In a varying proportion of cases (1% to 3%) symptoms may be aggravated. This seems to make little difference to the eventual recovery of the patient.
- Generalised reactions after treatment also occur, ranging from a pleasant drowsiness to disabling weakness and lethargy. Patients may also occasionally react severely during the treatment, with events such as fainting. Cancer patients are often more sensitive to acupuncture than other patients and many become excessively drowsy during treatment. It is advisable to have nursing assistance present, or assistance immediately available.
- Symptoms such as headache, nausea and vomiting, and dizziness can occur.

Patients are often cachectic and they should be given superficial needling with the greatest of care especially over the chest wall. It is unsafe to use acupuncture without a reasonably full knowledge of the clinical stage of the disease and the current status of orthodox therapy. (Filshie, 2001)

## 16.4 Regulation and training

Western medical acupuncture training is provided largely by the British Medical Acupuncture Society (BMAS) with a formal accreditation and reaccreditation process. Physiotherapists and nurses are trained on courses recognised by the Acupuncture Association of Chartered Physiotherapists, or the British Academy of Western Acupuncture. The British Medical Acupuncture Society offers specific foundation courses for doctors wanting to practise acupuncture in palliative care, and a supplementary one day course is also available for all practitioners who use acupuncture in palliative care.

Traditional acupuncturists, who may or may not be physicians, have undertaken a three year training course (or equivalent) accredited by the British Acupuncture Accreditation Board and are members of the professional body, the British Acupuncture Council. Traditional acupuncturists who have trained in other countries or on other courses can apply to the British Acupuncture Council admissions committee for validation of their qualification and practice in order to be eligible for registration with the British Acupuncture Council.

For information on regulation and national occupational standards, see Chapter 5 on regulation and training.

# 17 Homeopathy

## 17.1 Brief description

The word homeopathy comes from Greek and means similar suffering. It is the treatment of illness by using medication (known as remedies) prescribed according to the principle that 'like cures like'. That is to say, the patient is prescribed a remedy which, from experiment and experience, is known to produce very similar symptoms, when proved (tested) in healthy people, to the symptoms from which the patient is suffering.

The remedies used are derived from plant, animal and mineral sources which, through a process of serial dilution and agitation (succussion), are rendered dilute. (Lewith & Kenyon 2001; Thompson & Reilly 2002a) Homeopathy is not necessarily free of side effects, but a comprehensive search of the literature shows these to be rare, mild and transient. (Dantas & Rampes 2000) It is not possible to overdose on homeopathic medicines, in the usual understanding of the word, but taking more than one needs over a prolonged period can result in a proving of the remedy, which means that one starts to feel and exhibit the symptoms the remedy is meant to cure or relieve. These symptoms resolve when the remedy is stopped or changed to a more appropriate one.

There are different approaches to the practice of homeopathy. In the classical approach, one remedy is prescribed at a time, based on a match of one of the known remedy pictures to the patient's whole symptom picture, including the symptoms of their presenting or diagnosed complaint. Pluralist homeopathy involves the prescription of several single remedies at a time or close together, often in alternation, according to the practitioner's perception of different facets of the patient's condition that need to be treated. Complex homeopathy involves the use of fixed combinations of several remedies in single dose forms prescribed according to the conventional diagnosis of the patient's presenting condition. Some practitioners will use just one of these approaches while others may use a combination of them.

Homeopathy is practised by statutorily registered health care professionals, who have completed postgraduate studies in homeopathy and by other professional homeopaths. For many of the latter group, homeopathy is a second career, and they will often have other professional skills and expertise. The former group includes doctors, dentists, nurses and pharmacists who use their clinical judgement, within the clinical context in which they work, to determine the extent to which homeopathy is relevant to their patients; their training to use homeopathy builds on their primary professional training and expertise, and affiliation is to their primary profession. (*National Occupational Standards for Homeopathy*, Healthwork UK 2000)

## 17.2 Evidence

There have been several meta-analyses and systematic reviews of the use of homeopathy for different conditions, which show a positive trend, that homeopathy appears to be more effective than placebo (Kleijnen et al 1991; Linde, Melchart et al 1997; Linde & Melchart 1998, Cucherat, Boissel et al 2000). However, the conclusion is that the evidence is not sufficiently convincing for any one condition because of methodological shortcomings and inconsistencies, as well as some publication bias. The conclusion is that there is a need for more trials of greater methodological quality. It is also not known whether homeopathy is better than other standard treatments (as opposed to placebo), and for what conditions homeopathy is most effective. (RLHH 1999; Lewith & Kenyon 2001)

It was also recommended that homeopaths should critically evaluate their performance and personal experiences in well-planned case series and observational studies as clinical trials seemed to rarely reflect what happens in everyday practice. Homeopathic consultations, the review of cases and prescribing of remedies, involves consideration of the person as a whole and is highly individualised; this approach does not necessarily lend itself to clinical research.

Ernst's (1999) systematic review of trials of classical homeopathy versus conventional medications for adults and children with rheumatoid arthritis, proctocolitis, irritable bowel disease, malaria, otitis media or tonsillitis, found that the few comparative clinical trials of homeopathy contain serious methodological flaws. He concludes that the value of homeopathy compared to allopathic medication is unknown. However, Ernst's (2001) overview of exemplary studies and available systematic reviews of complementary therapies in palliative care concluded that, although the evidence is not compelling for any of the therapies, promising results exist for some treatments, including homeopathy.

Since the above reviews were published, there have been other randomised controlled trials. A double blind randomised controlled trial on the efficacy of homeopathic treatment for skin reactions during radiotherapy following surgery for breast cancer involved 65 women. (Balzarini, Felisi & De Canno 2000) The results suggested that the homeopathic complex was superior to a placebo in minimising the dermatological adverse effects of radiotherapy. Plans for a Cochrane review of homeopathy for cancer is underway. (Kassab et al 2003)

Oberbaum (1998) described the use of a homeopathic complex preparation in chemotherapy induced stomatitis in an uncontrolled study with 27 patients, and found a reduction in the duration of symptoms in the treated group. This study was followed by a randomised, double blind controlled trial of the homeopathic medication TRAUMEEL S[3] in the treatment of chemotherapy induced stomatitis in 32 children undergoing stem cell transplant. (Oberbaum et al 2001) Stomatitis scores were evaluated according to the World Health Organisation grading system for mucositis. Results indicated that TRAUMEEL S may reduce significantly the severity and duration of chemotherapy induced stomatitis in children undergoing bone marrow transplantation. The results of this study are being taken forward in a multi-centre trial on the use of TRAUMEEL S in adults undergoing bone marrow transplant. (Thompson 2002)

There are a number of outcome based observational studies which support the use of homeopathy in cancer care for psychological distress, including anxiety and depression (Clover, Fisher et al 1995), pain (Vozianov & Simeonova 1997, cited Thompson 1999), symptom control and its impact on mood disturbance and quality of life (Thompson & Reilly 2002a; Thompson & Reilly 2000b). A double blind randomised placebo-controlled trial of homeopathy in the management of menopausal symptoms in breast cancer survivors followed the above pilot study (Thompson & Reilly 2002b) and a paper on the study awaits publication. (Thompson 2003)

Good quality observational studies in various conditions including upper respiratory tract infections (Riley, Fisher et al 2001; Frei and Thurneysen 2001a), attention deficit hyperactivity disorder (Frei and Thurneysen 2001b), and headache (Muscari, Tomaioli et al 2001) consistently give positive results.

Case studies describe the effectiveness of homeopathy for various symptoms. These include the value of intrathecal baclofen and homeopathy for the treatment of painful muscle spasms associated with malignant spinal cord compression (Thompson

& Hicks 1998), and the use of homeopathic remedies for a patient with advanced cancer of the liver, spleen and gall bladder. (Every 1999)

Surveys of patient satisfaction and effectiveness from the patient's perspective of homeopathy used within a package of care showed high levels of satisfaction (Reilly 1995; Sharples & Van Haselen 1998; GHH 1998; Spene 1999 cited Boyd 2002; Ward 1994; Christie & Ward 1996). The surveys also showed a reduction in the use of conventional medication, an improvement in the presenting complaint, overall ability to cope and well-being, fewer appointments with the general practitioner, outpatients and admissions to other hospitals.

In summary, the evidence for the clinical effectiveness of homeopathy is mixed (Lewith & Kenyon 2001), and scientific research into homeopathy in the cancer setting is in its infancy (Thompson & Reilly 2002). Nevertheless, homeopathy is used by cancer patients (Downer et al 1994) and there is evidence that patients find the approach helpful. Homeopathy is available on the NHS, mainly through the five homeopathic hospitals in London, Bristol, Glasgow, Liverpool and Tunbridge Wells. Although more detailed clinical research is required, the best available evidence suggests that there is some basis for prescribing homeopathic remedies in the following circumstances:

- **Fatigue** (Thompson & Reilly 2002a and b)
- **Hot flushes** (Thompson & Reilly 2002a and b)
- **Pain, including joint pain and muscle spasm** (Clover, Fisher et al 1995; Vozianov & Simeonova 1997; Thompson & Hicks 1998; Thompson & Reilly 2002a)
- **Anxiety and stress** (Clover, Fisher et al 1995;Thompson & Reilly 2002a and b)
- **Depression** (Thompson & Reilly 2002a and b)
- **Quality of life, including mood disturbance** (Clover, Fisher, et al 1995; Thompson & Reilly 2002 and b)
- **Radiotherapy and skin reactions** (Balzarini, Felisi & De Canno 2000)
- **Post-surgery ileus** (Barnes, Resch & Ernst 1997)

3 TRAUMEEL S is a homeopathic complex remedy that has been sold over the counter in pharmacies in Germany, Austria and Switzerland for over 50 years. It contains extracts from the following plants and minerals, all of them highly diluted (10-1 – 10-9 of the stem solution): Arnica montana, Calendula officinalis, Achillea millefolium, Matricaria chamomilla, Symphytum officinale, Atropa belladonna, Aconitum napellus, Bellis perennis, Hypericum perforatum, Echinacea angustifolia, Echinacea purpurea, Hamamelis virginica, Mercurius solubilis and Hepar sulfuris. Information from the manufacturer indicates that TRAUMEEL S is used normally to treat trauma, inflammation and degenerative processes.

## 17.3 The use of homeopathy in supportive and palliative care

Precautions (Scrine 2002; Thompson & Reilly 2002a; Fisher 2003)
The reviews of the safety of homeopathy conclude that the main risks are indirect rather than direct, that is they relate to practitioners, not the medicines.

- **Be aware** that aggravation of symptoms at the start of treatment is unusual in palliative care, is usually short-term and falls away gradually.
- **Be aware** of aggravation of symptoms following repeated doses of a remedy. Homeopaths will usually stop the remedy or decrease the frequency of administration, which should be accompanied by an overall improvement in well-being within a couple of weeks.
- **Be aware** that a return of old symptoms is thought to be a response of the body's self-healing mechanism. In the process of positive change, previous trauma is revisited briefly before an overall improvement is experienced
- **Be aware** that new symptoms may mean that the remedy does not match the patient's symptoms and needs to be changed. This can also occur if the correct remedy is chosen but is given too frequently, or if the patient has a history of sensitivity to other medication. When the remedy is stopped, symptoms should cease.
- **Be aware** of possible effects on symptom control and conventional medication. If homeopathic remedies reduce pain or improve other symptoms, the dose of allopathic medication may need to be reviewed. Otherwise, the clinical experience of homeopaths is that homeopathic remedies are unlikely to interact with allopathic medication in the usual chemical understanding of the term.
- **Be aware** of practitioners' lack of understanding of disease process and treatment
- **Be aware** of practitioners' lack of awareness of the bounds of their own competence

## 16.4 Regulation and training

### Training
Statutorily regulated health care professionals mostly undertake their post-graduate homeopathy studies with the Faculty of Homeopathy. There are a number of private and university educated homeopaths who are voluntarily self-regulated. The Council of Organisations Registering Homeopaths (CORH) consists of organisations that register homeopaths. The Faculty of Homeopathy and the Council of Organisations Registering Homeopaths agree that education and training should enable all homeopaths who practise independently, to practise at the level of the national occupational standards for homeopathy (Healthwork UK 2000).

At the Faculty of Homeopathy, there is a structured three level training pathway for medical homeopaths, to licentiate (one year introductory, LFHom), membership (after 4-5 years, MFHom), and specialist register level (a further 2-3 years). The different levels of training qualify doctors for different levels of practice. The completion of the membership level training certifies a doctor's competence to use homeopathy in a wide range of clinical situations in primary care or on referral, with the support of specialist colleagues. A further two years' specialist training qualifies a doctor for independent specialist practice in the community or within a medical speciality. The diploma level is for dentists and pharmacists (DFHom).

For other professional homeopaths education and training is delivered either through three year full-time or four year part-time courses in private educational institutions or through university based degree courses. The University of Westminster and University of Central Lancashire currently offer three year full-time BSc (Hons) degree courses of education and training in homeopathy.

### Licence to practise
Statutorily regulated health care practitioners who practise homeopathy carry a statutory licence to practise by virtue of their registration with their relevant regulatory body.

Other professional homeopaths are granted diplomas or university degrees together with a licence to practise by their educational establishment once they have successfully completed the course. Although the licence to practise is not a legal requirement and does not have any legal status, the courses accepted by the professional bodies define the terms on which a licence to practise can be awarded to students. They further stipulate the terms on which candidates can proceed to a register.

### Regulation
Information on the regulation of homeopaths can be found in Chapter 5 on regulation and training.

# 18 Guideline development process

## 18.1 Steering group

The steering group for the project was drawn from major stakeholding organisations and professionals within palliative care, service users and representatives from a range of service delivery organisations.

Michael Fox, (joint chair) Chief Executive, The Prince of Wales's Foundation for Integrated Health

Eve Richardson, (joint chair) Chief Executive, National Council for Hospice and Specialist Palliative Care Services

Marianne Tavares, Project Manager, Complementary Therapies in Palliative Care, The Prince of Wales's Foundation for Integrated Health

Judy Abbott, service user, Sheffield

Angela Avis MBE,Chair, Complementary Therapies Forum, Royal College of Nursing; Lecturer, Oxford Brookes University

Ann Carter, Complementary Therapy Co-ordinator, St. Ann's Hospice, Manchester

Liz Hawkins, Complementary Therapy Co-ordinator, St. Christopher's Hospice (until Sept 2002); Lecturer, University of Westminster; Complementary Therapy Practitioner, Harley Street Clinic

Jean Hindmarch, Head of Education, Training and Awards, Help the Hospices

Dr. Jenny Kitchen, Consultant in Palliative Medicine, The Shropshire and Mid Wales Hospice, (until July 2002), St. Peter's Hospice, Bristol (from July 2002)

Dr. Michelle Kohn, Complementary Therapies Medical Adviser, Macmillan Cancer Relief

Peter Mackereth, Lecturer/Practitioner in Complementary Therapies (from March 2002), Christie Hospital NHS Trust, Manchester; Lecturer, Salford University

Freda Magee, Chair, (from June 2002) National Association of Complementary Therapists in Hospice and Palliative Care

Dr. Andrew Manasse, Clinical Lead, The Cavendish Centre for Cancer Care, Sheffield

John Pickett, service user, London

Jan Wilkinson, Vice Chair, (until June 2002) National Association of Complementary Therapists in Hospice and Palliative Care

Dr. Susie Wilkinson, Head of Caring Services Research, Marie Curie Palliative Care RND Unit; Senior Lecturer, Department of Oncology, Royal Free University College Medical School

## 18.2 Gathering information and evidence

### Existing guidelines, policies and standards

500 organisations, as listed in the Directory of Hospice and Palliative Care Services, 2001, were approached for their existing guidelines, policies and standards with regard to complementary therapies. Policies were received from about 100 organisations. Another 20 replied that they either did not offer complementary therapies, or were currently developing or updating their policies.

The most widely provided therapies, and issues addressed in local policies were identified from the sets of guidelines received. Using the information provided, a draft outline of the national guidelines was drawn up, and sent to the wider consultative group for the project.

### Consulting professional organisations for complementary therapies

The professional organisations for massage, aromatherapy, reflexology, acupuncture, homeopathy, hypnotherapy, and healing were invited to contribute to the development process. Contacts were identified through the regulation programme of The Prince of Wales's Foundation for Integrated Health, and the following information was requested:
- Brief description
- Evidence base, especially for palliative care
- How patients can benefit from use of the therapy in palliative care
- General contraindications and precautions for the therapy
- Specific contraindications and precautions for using the therapy in palliative care
- Modification of approach in palliative care
- Other issues for consideration
- Practitioner training and qualification, regulatory bodies

## 18.3 Consultation and peer review

### Symposia

Three symposia were held in London, Bristol and Manchester, involving about 100 service users and professionals with responsibility for developing complementary therapy services. Services users were approached via Cancerlink, and professionals were invited from a range of providers including hospitals, hospices, and cancer support centres in different parts of England and Wales. The experience of service providers ranged from those in the early stages of developing complementary therapy services to centres of excellence. Appendix M gives the list of participants in the three symposia. The symposia identified important areas for inclusion in the guidelines.

### Experts

Drafts of the relevant sections were sent to different experts and experienced practitioners of the therapy within supportive and palliative care (see Appendix O). Some experts contributed to the writing of the drafts.

### National consultation

The national consultation process for the draft document was as follows:

- Publication of the draft document on the websites of The Prince of Wales's Foundation for Integrated Health www.fihealth.org.uk and the National Council for Hospice and Specialist Palliative Care Services www.hospice-spc-council.org.uk
- Distribution of the document to the participants of the symposia (Appendix M), the professional bodies for the therapies included in the guidelines, the wider consultative group (Appendix N), the list of experts (Appendix O), and as requested.

### External Evaluation

There will be a process for evaluating the usefulness of the guidelines following publication, led by Professor Jessica Corner. The guidelines will be disseminated to palliative care organisations from whom feedback is also welcomed.

# 19 Appendices

## Appendix A
## Configuration of Complementary Therapy Teams: Models of Service Provision

**A 1** Cancer Support Centre
The Cavendish Centre for Cancer Care, Sheffield

Founded in 1992; charitable organisation, offering assessment, support and a range of complementary therapies to patients at all stages of disease, integrated with their NHS care. Services are patient centred and patient led, include children and carers, and are free of charge. Patients self refer, and are seen usually within 5 working days. Patient care is audited using an established outcome measure.

| | |
|---|---|
| Director | • Overall responsibility for: all aspects of the centre's activity; the running of the centre; forward planning<br>• Heads the management team and is accountable to the trustees |
| Clinical lead, currently a doctor (this role is changing - there is currently considerable overlap with the new therapy services manager's role) | • On management team<br>• Oversees research, issues related to provision of therapy, relationship with NHS professionals especially medical profession, teaching<br>• Answers therapy related questions from the public |
| Therapy services manager<br>(This is a new post; there is considerable overlap with the existing clinical lead role which is changing) | • On management team<br>• Assessment, co-ordination and management of clinical services<br>• Responsible for service development<br>• Provision of support for clinical staff<br>• Ensures effective communication between clinical staff<br>• Teaching and developing links with other health care professionals working in cancer care |
| Assessors/key workers | • Provide a key role in the process; overall responsibility for the patient's pathway through the centre; close relationship with therapists<br>• Assess patient/carer needs and decide most appropriate therapy, with client<br>• Communicate routinely with all healthcare professionals involved with the patient/carer<br>• Review client following course of therapy, carried out by same assessor who originally assessed the client<br>• Manage outcome evaluation<br>• Involved in running carer and bereavement groups |
| Complementary therapists, all self-employed | • Provide time limited courses of therapy: acupuncture, aromatherapy, art therapy, counselling, healing, homeopathy, hypnotherapy, massage, reflexology, relaxation/visualisation, shiatsu and herbal medicine<br>• Some take part in running groups<br>• Responsible for own therapy specific professional support and for continuing professional development<br>• Have own professional indemnity |
| Fundraiser | • On management team<br>• Responsible for all aspects of fundraising<br>• Accountable to director |
| Office manager, a key post within the organisation | • Member of management team<br>• Manages general office and reception – responsible for smooth running and appearance of Centre<br>• Manages all financial transactions for the Centre |
| Receptionists, a very important first contact point | • Receive all incoming calls from patients<br>• Welcome people who drop in, and patients coming for appointments, including offering refreshments<br>• Introduce the Centre to patients, give information<br>• Make appointments |

| Volunteer development manager | • Recruits, trains, manages, supports and retains 60 volunteers<br>• Develops volunteer projects, teams and individuals<br>• Member of management team<br>• Represents centre at forums/arenas related to volunteers through the city |
|---|---|
| Volunteers (do not provide therapy) | • Many different activities: charity shop, fundraising events, reception and office support, website design, editing internal and external newsletters, organising and distributing information and newsletters, speaking to community groups |

## A 2 Hospital Complementary Therapy Team

Hammersmith Hospitals NHS Trust, Cancer Services Complementary Therapy Team, London
The service operates across the two sites of Charing Cross and Hammersmith Hospitals, within cancer services – outpatients and inpatients receiving treatment, eg radiotherapy chemotherapy and symptom control. There is also staff massage

| Complementary therapy team leader, permanent contract (nursing budget)<br><br>Deputy team leader, permanent contract (nursing budget) | • Responsible for service development, including development of policy and protocols, documentation, evaluation of service<br>• Manages the service, including recruitment, referral and appointments system<br>• Manages therapy team, and provides supervision<br>• Provides therapies<br>• Contributes to the in-house education and training of staff with cancer services<br>• Provides supervision for massage students doing clinical placements at both hospitals |
|---|---|
| Complementary therapists, permanent contracts (nursing budget) | • Provide aromatherapy, massage, reflexology, relaxation, visualisation and art therapy |
| Complementary therapists, self-employed honorary contracts (oncology budget and other funds) | • Provide aromatherapy, reflexology and massage |
| Nurses and health care assistants with a qualification in massage or reflexology, who have undergone training with the complementary therapy team, and who are allocated time by their ward manager | • Provide massage and reflexology within their working week to treat patients on their ward |
| Student massage therapists, (placements) undergraduates and post-graduates | • Provide massage, mainly feet and hands |

## A 3 Hospital Rehabilitation Team

The Royal Marsden Hospital, London and Sutton
For cancer services, inpatients and outpatients in rehabilitation unit and wards

| Rehabilitation centre manager | • Provides overall strategic direction and management<br>• Responsible for resource allocation<br>• Responsible for co-ordination of service within rehabilitation |
|---|---|
| Nurse consultant in cancer care (Rehabilitation) | Function with respect to complementary therapies:<br>• Overall responsibility for service development, standard setting, audit, policy development and research<br>• Works with complementary therapy team leader and other health care professionals to develop services collaboratively |

| Complementary therapy team leader | • Provides massage and aromatherapy<br>• Manages other therapists<br>• Works with nurse consultant to develop policies, training and documentation |
| --- | --- |
| Complementary therapists | • Provide massage and aromatherapy |
| Nurses | • Use therapy skills alongside nursing role with inpatients, following in-house training |

NB  Additionally, acupuncture is provided on both hospital sites and given by consultant anaesthetists for pain and symptom control in a multidisciplinary setting.

## A 4 NHS Specialist Complementary Medicine Hospital

The Royal London Homoeopathic Hospital, part of University College London Hospitals NHS Trust
Provides packages of a range of complementary medicine therapies for various conditions. Complementary cancer care is one of the larger services.

• Founded in 1849 and part of the NHS since its inception.
• Takes referrals from all over England and Wales (mostly London and SE England) from GPs or hospital/hospice specialists.
• Cancer treatments are offered on an outpatient, daycare or inpatient basis and include homoeopathy, Iscador, acupuncture, aromatherapy massage, reflexology, reiki, shiatsu, relaxation and visualisation.
• All homeopaths and therapists are statutorily regulated healthcare professionals with additional training in complementary medicine.
• Cross referral to other RLHH services, not mentioned below, as required.
• Treatments are designed to complement conventional cancer care with ongoing liaison between RLHH and the patient's healthcare professionals.

| Director of complementary cancer services | • Overall responsibility for service development, research and audit<br>• Screens all new referrals letters and directs to appropriate doctor/clinic<br>• Provides homeopathy, Iscador, acupuncture on outpatient, daycare or inpatient basis<br>• Provides education to healthcare professionals on complementary medicine for cancer |
| --- | --- |
| Homeopathic physicians | • Provide homeopathy, Iscador and acupuncture on an outpatient basis |
| Nurse and therapies manager | • Responsibility for developing nurse therapists<br>• Oversees delivery and audit of nurse therapies<br>• Clinical supervision<br>• Teaches autogenic training, relaxation, lifestyle management<br>• Provides aromatherapy massage and reflexology |
| Nurse therapists | • Provide aromatherapy massage, reflexology, shiatsu, reiki, relaxation and TCM acupuncture |
| Access to state registered dietician | • Dietary review and appropriate, sensible nutritional advice |
| Access to autogenic trainers | • For relief of stress and anxiety |

## A 5 Hospice Complementary Therapies Service
### St. Gemma's Hospice, Leeds

Specialist palliative care unit, inpatient unit with 32 beds, day hospice, community team. For inpatients, outpatients, day hospice patients, carers and staff

| | |
|---|---|
| Complementary therapies coordinator, permanent contract (within budget for allied health professionals) | • Responsible for service development, including development of policy and protocols, documentation, evaluation of service<br>• Manages the service, including recruitment, referral and appointments system, equipment<br>• Manages other therapists and provides supervision<br>• Provides massage, aromatherapy and reiki<br>• Provides training for therapy assistants |
| Complementary therapists (self-employed) | • Provide massage, aromatherapy and reiki<br>• Supports therapy assistants |
| Volunteer complementary therapists | • Provide massage, aromatherapy, reiki and acupuncture |
| Other members of clinical team (nurses, health care assistants, social worker, chaplains) | • Use therapy skills following suitable training (some in-house, some external) eg simple massage and reiki |
| Access to occupational therapist, physiotherapist | • For assessment and therapy/aids as required |
| Access to social worker team | • For counselling |
| Access to other members of multidisciplinary team | • For review and to integrate care |

## A 6 Multi-site Hospice and Cancer Support Centre

For inpatients, outpatients, day hospice patients
St. Ann's Hospice, incorporating Neil Cliffe Cancer Care Centre (rehab unit) and sites at Heald Green and Little Hulton in Greater Manchester

Complementary therapy is regarded as core business and has an integral role to play in the care of patients and their carers. The service is well-established and offers a variety of approaches to help with the relief of stress, anxiety and tension.

| | |
|---|---|
| Complementary therapy co-ordinator (Part time 22.5 hours per week ) | • Has responsibility for the co-ordination and development of the Complementary Therapy Service across the three sites. |
| On the hospice sites, any health care professional may refer a patient/carer for complementary therapy.<br><br>Key workers (professional backgrounds of nursing, at rehabilitation unit only) | • Assesses patient needs, agrees goals and decides with the patient a plan of action. Patient choice is from a wide range of services of which complementary therapy is just one.<br>The number of sessions is agreed with the patient, up to four sessions initially. Review takes place at end of the agreed number of sessions |
| Complementary therapists may be:<br>• self employed on a sessional basis<br>• nurses on either hospice site<br>• other health care professionals e.g doctors, physiotherapists with an appropriate qualification | • On each of the hospice sites therapists offer: aromatherapy, reflexology and reiki and Indian head massage.<br>• The benefits of essential oils and bases in wound care are being explored on the two hospice sites<br>• Hypnotherapy and neurolinguistic programming is also used as part of the role of the psychological support nurse<br>• At the Neil Cliffe Cancer Care Centre acupuncture, craniosacral therapy, homeopathy and therapeutic massage are also offered in addition to aromotherapy, reflexology and reiki. |

- A special clinic also combines the skills of a physiotherapist and an aromatherapist to help patients who mainly experience problems associated with breast cancer.
- The Neil Cliffe Centre also hosts a "Stress Busters" service which offers therapies to staff and the public one evening per week.

| Health care professionals, mainly nurses and care assistants | • Use hands on therapeutic skills following house training for the "HEARTS" process. This approach was devised to extend the therapeutic use of touch for therapists and health care professionals. In house training is given to acquire the skills. |
| --- | --- |

## A 7 Self-Help Group
## Northumberland Cancer Support Group (affiliated to Bristol Cancer Help Centre)

Founded in 1986; a committee of volunteers runs the group. The committee works as a team: many tasks overlap; annual planning and review session; varied programme of activities, including discussion nights, fun nights, gentle yoga, circle dancing, guest speakers, complementary therapies, social events; whole group meets weekly on Tuesday evenings

Complementary therapies are offered free-of-charge at weekly meetings, at home and in hospital. Priority is given to members in greatest need

| Chair | • Chairs monthly committee meetings<br>• Deals with condolence letters<br>• Purchases, then sells to the group vitamins and minerals as recommended by the Bristol Cancer Help Centre |
| --- | --- |
| Secretary | • Responsible for minutes of committee meetings, and other correspondence<br>• Does a great deal of typing and photocopying, and orders stationery<br>• Updates members and non-members mailing list<br>• Organises distribution of information, including the programme of events, to members<br>• Compiles and contacts people taking part in the group programme<br>• A telephone contact for people seeking support and information |
| Treasurer | • Oversees expenditure<br>• Responsible for accounts and banking<br>• Issues cheques<br>• Arranges annual audit |
| Publicity coordinator | • Assists secretary, especially with photocopying<br>• Distributes leaflets and other information in hospitals, surgeries, clinics and other public places<br>• Collates a data bank of contacts re information<br>• Organises information in the press<br>• Assists with fundraising events |
| Volunteer coordinator | • Organises training for volunteers and therapists (weekend training workshops and external supervision sessions are held regularly for volunteers)<br>• Organises volunteer and therapist meetings<br>• Liaises with care co-ordinator regarding home/hospital visits<br>• Compiles and distributes a therapist rota |
| Care coordinator | • Identifies those members of the group who need particular support and help.<br>• Discusses issues involved with the committee, and oversees actions to be taken by the committee<br>• Collates information regarding attendance<br>• One of three telephone contacts for people seeking support and information |

| | |
|---|---|
| | • Arranges home and hospital visits by volunteers and therapists<br>• Active in all fundraising events |
| Librarian | • Organises the running of the library<br>• Reviews and updates the books, cassettes and videos in the library<br>• Deals with the purchase of new stock<br>• Supervises the training of library assistants<br>• Supervises the library rota |
| Fundraising coordinators (2) | • Organise fundraising events<br>• Delegate jobs to committee and group members<br>• Deal with publicity regarding events<br>• Apply for grants and donations |
| Complementary therapists<br>(all volunteers, qualified and insured) | • Provide gentle massage, reflexology, reiki, Indian head massage, shiatsu, aromatherapy, counselling<br>• Provide treatment at weekly meetings, at home and in hospitals |

## Appendix B
## Main components of clinical governance (Department of Health 1999)

**1. Clear lines of responsibility and accountability for the overall quality of clinical care**

This is achieved through formally designated individuals, as well as regular and annual reports.

**2. A comprehensive programme of quality improvement activities which includes:**
- Full participation in audit programmes
- Full participation in the national confidential enquiries
- Evidence-based practice which is supported and applied routinely in everyday practice
- Ensuring the clinical standards of national service frameworks and NICE recommendations are implemented
- Workforce planning and development such as recruitment and retention of appropriately trained workforce is fully integrated within the NHS organisation's service planning
- Continuing professional development: programmes aimed at meeting the development needs of individual health professionals and the service needs of the organisation are in place and supported locally
- Appropriate safeguards to govern access to and storage of confidential patient information as recommended in the Caldicott Report on Review of Patient-Identifiable Information
- Effective monitoring of clinical care with high quality systems for clinical record keeping and the collection of relevant information
- Processes for assuring the quality of clinical care are in place and integrated with the quality programme for the organisation as a whole
- Participation in well-designed relevant research and development activity is encouraged and supported as something which can contribute to the development of an 'evaluation culture'.

**3. Clear policies aimed at managing risks:**
- Controls assurance which promote self assessment to identify and manage risks
- Clinical risk systematically assessed with programmes in place to reduce risk

**4. Procedures for all professional groups to identify and remedy poor performance, for example:**
- Critical incident reporting ensures that adverse events are identified, openly investigated, lessons are learned and promptly applied
- Complaints procedures, accessible to patients and their families and fair to staff. Lessons are learned and recurrence of similar problems avoided
- Professional performance procedures which take effect at an early stage before patients are harmed and which help the individual to improve their performance whenever possible, are in place and understood by all staff
- Staff supported in their duty to report any concerns about colleagues' professional conduct and performance, with clear statements on what is expected of all staff. Clear procedures for reporting concerns so that early action can be taken to remedy the situation

# Appendix C
## Resources for conducting audit, evaluation and research

### Books

Bowling A. *Measuring Health: a review of quality of life measurement scales*. 2nd edition. Open University Press, Buckingham, 1997

Lewith G, Jonas WB, Walach H. (editors). *Clinical Research in Complementary Therapies: principles, problems and solutions*. Churchill Livingstone, London 2002

### Advice and information

Lesley Foulkes (re: the Practice Based Health Outcome Measure)
Newcastle Homeopathic Practice
The Light House
18 Water Street
Newcastle
Staffordshire ST5 1JQ
Tel. 01782 633759
Email: lfoulkes@homeopathy-soh.org

On MYCAW and MYMOP questionnaires (see Paterson 2000 and Paterson 2002)
Dr. Charlotte Paterson
MRC Health Services Research Collaboration
Department of Social Medicine, University of Bristol
Canynge Hall
Whiteladies Road
Bristol BS8 2PR
Email: C.Paterson@bristol.ac.uk

Dr. Kate Thomas
Senior Lecturer in Health Services Research;
Deputy Director, Medical Care Research Unit
ScHARR
University of Sheffield
Regent Court
30 Regent Street
Sheffield S1 4DA
Tel. 0114 222 0753 /0114 222 5202
Email k.j.thomas@sheffield.ac.uk

Dr. E.A. Thompson
Chair: Regional Complementary Therapy Research Group
Consultant Homeopathic Physician and Honorary Senior Lecturer in Palliative Care
Bristol Homeopathic Hospital
Cotham Hill
Bristol BS6 6JU
Tel. 0117 973 1231
Fax 0117 923 8759
Email: elizabeth.thompson@ubht.swest.nhs.uk

Dr. Susie Wilkinson
Head of Caring Services Research, Senior Lecturer
Marie Curie Palliative Care R&D Unit
Department of Oncology
Royal Free University College Medical School
Royal Free Campus
Rowland Hill Street
London NW3 2PF
Email: swilkinson@rfc.ucl.ac.uk

### Health services research units:
Contact school of health care studies of nearest university

**The Cavendish Centre for Cancer Care**
27 Wilkinson Street
Sheffield
South Yorkshire S10 2GB
Tel. 0114 278 4600
Email: enquiries@cavcare.org

**National Association of Complementary Therapists in Hospice and Palliative Care**
29 King's Road
Berkhamsted
Herts HP4 3BH
Tel. 01442 874226
Email: nacthpc@hotmail.com

**The Prince of Wales's Foundation for Integrated Health**
12 Chillingworth Road
London N7 8QJ
Tel. 020 7619 6140
Fax 020 7700 8434
Email: info@fihealth.org.uk
Website: www.fihealth.org.uk

**The Research Council for Complementary Medicine**
27a Devonshire Street
London W1G 6PN
Tel. 020 7935 7499
Fax. 020 7935 2460
Email: info@rccm.org.uk
Website: www.rccm.org.uk
For good basic information on research and clinical audit

## Appendix D
## Evidence for best practice
(Richardson 2001)

Important electronic databases that include articles and research information on complementary therapies

### AMED (Alternative and Allied Medicine Database)
Database established in 1985 by the British Library's Medical Information Centre. Total of 65,000 references. Scans 400 journals for references to complementary therapy. Also contains references for physiotherapy, occupational therapy, rehabilitation and podiatry. Updated monthly. Access by licence only, usually available in NHS libraries

### CAM on PubMed (Medline)
Developed jointly by NIH Centre for Complementary and Alternative Medicine and the National Library of Medicine.
www.nlm.nih.gov/nccam/camonpubmed.html

### CISCOM (The Centralised Information Service for Complementary Medicine)
Specialist information service based on a database produced by the Research Council for Complementary Medicine. Contains around 70,000 references. Combines data from a wide range of sources including in house citation tracking. A specialist thesaurus is currently being developed. Specialises in clinical trials. Also holds references to sociological and psychological studies.
www.rccm.org.uk

### Complementary Medicine Programme Database
A programme that facilitates systematic reviews and evaluation. Includes the complementary and alternative medicine and pain database (CAMPAIN)
www.compmed.ummc.umaryland.edu/default.htm

### HerbMed
Herbal database that provides hyperlinked access to the scientific data underlying the use of herbs. An evidence based information resource for professionals, researchers and general public. Contains 125 evidence based reviews of herbal therapies.
www.herbmed.org/

### Hom-Inform information service
Contains 17,000 references based on contents of Faculty of Homoeopathy library based at Glasgow Homoeopathic Hospital
hominform.soutron.com/homqbe1.asp

### BNI (British Nursing Index)
Has a nursing focus but with some complementary therapy references. Access by licence only, usually available in NHS libraries

### Cinahl (Cumulative Index to Nursing and Allied Health Literature)
Records of literature on all aspects of nursing and allied health disciplines, includes some complementary therapy references. Access by licence only, usually available in NHS libraries

### NHS Centre for Reviews and Dissemination
Includes the DARE database, economic evaluation database and health technology programme reports.
www.york.ac.uk/inst/crd

### OMNI gateway
Provides free access to a searchable catalogue of internet sites covering health and medicine, including complementary medicine
http://omni.ac.uk

### Cochrane Reviews
Examples of published reviews:

Acupuncture for chronic asthma
www.update-software.com/abstracts/ab000008.htm

Acupuncture for induction of labour
www.update-software.com/abstracts/ab001218.htm

Alexander technique for chronic asthma
www.update-software.com/abstracts/ab000995.htm

Massage for promoting growth and development of pre-term and low birth-weight babies
www.update-software.com/abstracts/ab000390.htm

Massage for low back pain
www.update-software.com/abstracts/ab001929.htm

St. John's Wort for depression
www.update-software.com/abstracts/ab000448.htm

Yoga for epilepsy
www.update-software.com/abstracts/ab001524.htm

### Examples of reviews in progress:
Complementary therapies for acne
Gingko biloba in intermittent claudication
Massage and aromatherapy for symptom relief in patients with cancer
Mind body therapy for fibromyalgia
Reflexology for symptom relief in patients with cancer
Stress management for coronary heart disease
Therapeutic touch in wound healing

Information details:
Cochrane Library
The Cochrane Library contains over 5000 reports of randomised controlled trials and over 60 systematic reviews on complementary therapies (subscription required).
www.cochranelibrary.com/enter/

RCCM (Research Council for Complementary Medicine) website
Abstracts of the Cochrane Reviews of complementary therapy available on the RCCM website.
www.rccm.org.uk/cochrane.htm

Cochrane Complementary and Alternative Medicine Field
Registry of randomised controlled trials, located at the University of Maryland Complementary Medicine Programme
www.compmed.ummc.umaryland.edu/Compmed/ Cochrane/Cochrane.htm

## Appendix E
## Working groups developing single regulatory bodies, for the therapies included in these guidelines

### Acupuncture

| Working group | Members of working group | Development of national occupational standards (NOS) |
|---|---|---|
| Acupuncture Regulatory Working Group | • Acupuncture Association of Chartered Physiotherapists (AACP)<br>• British Academy of Western Acupuncture (BAWA)<br>• British Acupuncture Council (BAcC)<br>• British Medical Acupuncture Society (BMAS) | Agreed to develop NOS |

The Acupuncture Regulatory Working Group is working to develop recommendations for the statutory regulation of acupuncture in England, and its report is expected by July 2003. Acupuncture organisations not represented on the working group will be included in the consultation process. The Acupuncture Regulatory Working Group is supported by the Department of Health and The Prince of Wales's Foundation for Integrated Health. See also Chapter 16 for further information about the training of acupuncturists.

### Aromatherapy

| Working group | Members of working group | Development of national occupational standards |
|---|---|---|
| Aromatherapy Regulation Working Group | • Aromatherapy Organisations Council (AOC*)<br>• International Federation of Professional Aromatherapists (IFPA)<br>• Institute of Complementary Medicine (ICM/BRCP)<br>• British Complementary Medicine Association (BCMA)<br>• The Aromatherapists Society (AS)<br>• Professional Association of Clinical Therapists (PACT – part of Federation of Holistic Therapists) | Completed and published |
| | * Members of AOC<br>Aromatherapy & Allied Practitioner's Association (AAPA)<br>Association of Holistic Therapies Intl (AHPI)<br>Association of Medical Aromatherapists (AMA)<br>Association of Natural Medicine (ANM)<br>Association of Physical & Natural Therapists (APNT)<br>English Societe de L'Institute Pierre Franchome (ESIPF)<br>Intl Holistic Aromatherapy Foundations (IHA)<br>International Federation of Aromatherapists (IFA)<br>International Guild of Professional Practitioners<br>Renbardou Institute (RI) | |

## Homeopathy

| Working group | Members of working group | Development of national occupational standards |
|---|---|---|
| Council of Organisations Registering Homeopaths (CORH) | • Alliance of Registered Homeopaths (ARH)<br>• Assoc. of Natural Medicine<br>• Institute of Complementary Medicine (ICM/BRCP)<br>• Complementary Medical Association (CMA)<br>• Fellowship of Homeopaths (FoH)<br>• Homeopathic Medical Association (HMA)<br>• International Guild of Professional Practitioners<br>• Intl Register of Consultant Herbalists (IRCH)<br>• Society of Homeopaths (SoH) | Completed and published |

Statutorily regulated health care professionals who practise homeopathy can become members of the Faculty of Homeopathy. However, the Faculty is not a regulatory body, and these professionals are regulated by the regulatory body for their relevant profession. The Faculty of Homeopathy was involved in the development of national occupational standards for homeopathy. For information on the training of homeopaths, refer to Chapter 17 on homeopathy.

## Hypnosis and hypnotherapy

| Working group | Members of working group | Development of national occupational standards |
|---|---|---|
| Has not been agreed | N/A | 1st edition completed and published;<br>2nd edition in progress |

Professionals with a conventional health care qualification are trained to use hypnosis by the British Society of Medical and Dental Hypnosis, the British Society of Experimental and Clinical Hypnosis, and some university departments. Psychotherapists trained in hypnotherapy are registered with the United Kingdom Council for Psychotherapists.

Apart from the above, hypnotherapists are trained at a large number of other establishments. The level of training is varied and there is currently no agreed standard or core curriculum. For further information, refer to Chapter 15 on hypnosis and hypnotherapy.

## Massage Therapy

| Working group | Members of working group | Development of national occupational standards |
|---|---|---|
| General Council for Massage Therapy (GCMT) | • Fellowship of Sports Masseurs and Therapists (FSMT)<br>• International Guild of Professional Practitioners<br>• London & Counties Society of Physiologists (LCSP)<br>• Massage Therapy Institute of Great Britain (MTIGB)<br>• Massage Training Institute (MTI)<br>• Scottish Massage Therapists Organisation (SMTO)* | Draft in consultation, to be published in 2003 |

*Professional Association of Clinical Therapists (PACT, part of Federation of Holistic Therapists) have applied to join this working group.

Massage, as a manual therapy, is integral to the training of chartered physiotherapists. The Association of Chartered Physiotherapists in Massage can be contacted for further information  www.csp.org.uk

## Reiki

| Working group | Members of working group | Development of national occupational standards (NOS) |
| --- | --- | --- |
| UK Reiki Federation (UKRF) | The UKRF is making initial contact with a number of organisations to widen its remit. These include:<br>• The Reiki Association<br>• UK Reiki Alliance<br>• International Guild of Professional Practitioners<br>• Institute of Complementary Medicine (ICM/BRCP)<br>• British Complementary Medicine Association (BCMA) | UKRF have applied to develop NOS in the near future and have been involved in developing generic template for NOS in complementary therapies |

## Reflexology

| Working group | Members of working group | Development of national occupational standards |
| --- | --- | --- |
| Reflexology Forum | • Association of Reflexologists (AOR)<br>• British Reflexology Association (BRA)<br>• Centre for Clinical Reflexology (CCR)<br>• International Federation of Reflexologists (IFR)<br>• International Guild of Professional Practitioners<br>• International Institute of Reflexology (IIR)<br>• Reflexologists Society (RS)<br>• Reflexology Practitioners Association (RPA)<br>• Scottish Institute of Reflexology (SIR)<br>• Professional Association of Clinical Therapists (PACT, part of Federation of Holistic Therapists) | Completed and published |

The Association of Chartered Physiotherapists in Reflex Therapy can be contacted for further information on the use of reflexology by chartered physiotherapists within their scope of practice www.csp.org.uk

## Spiritual Healing

| Working group | Members of working group | Development of national occupational standards (NOS) |
| --- | --- | --- |
| UK Healers | • The Spiritualists National Union (SNU)<br>• The British Alliance of Healing Associations (BAHA)<br>• The World Federation of Healing (WFH)<br>• The School of Insight and Intuitions (School of Insight)<br>• Greater World Christian Spiritualist Associations (Greater World)<br>• White Rose Foundation (White Rose)<br>• Holistic Healers Association (Holistic Healers)<br>• White Eagle Lodge<br>• United Spiritualists<br>• National Federation of Spiritual Healers (NFSH)<br>• Northern Healers Forum (NHF)<br>• Confederation of Healing Organisations(CHO)<br>• Association of Therapeutic Healers (ATH) | UK Healers have applied to develop NOS in the near future and have been involved in developing a generic template for NOS in complementary therapies |

Therapeutic touch

| Working group | Members of working group | Development of national occupational standards |
|---|---|---|
| N/A | N/A | N/A |

Training courses for therapeutic touch, at practitioner level, are currently available in Lancaster, validated by St. Martin's College, University of Lancaster. Practitioners of therapeutic touch are currently registered with the British Association of Therapeutic Touch (BATT). For further information, refer to Chapter 14.5 on Therapeutic Touch, and visit the website www.sacredspace.org.uk

## Appendix F
# Sample job description for complementary therapies coordinator
(used with permission of St. Gemma's Hospice, Leeds)

### Job Description
Post: Complementary Therapies Co-ordinator
Accountable to: Chief Executive and Director of Nursing

Responsible to: Deputy Director of Nursing and Allied Health Professionals

St. Gemma's Hospice provides specialist palliative care to the population of Leeds and surrounding areas. The hospice has a large in-patient unit of 32 beds, a day hospice, hospice community team, out-patient service, education and conference centre, and a bereavement service.

### Primary Aim of Role
The Complementary Therapies Co-ordinator leads the development of complementary therapies and has a pivotal role in managing the provision of complementary therapies to inpatients, outpatients, day hospice and community patients, carers and staff.

- To communicate and work closely with all staff groups, particularly ward, day hospice and community teams.

- To be responsible for recruiting, managing and developing a team of qualified volunteer complementary therapists to work in palliative care.

- To identify needs in relation to the development of complementary therapies, and co-ordinate the introduction of other therapies.

- To collaborate with the Education Department, in particular the training and development of complementary therapy helpers.

- To address issues of quality, training, audit, research and development in complementary therapies.

### Main Responsibilities
#### 1 Clinical
1.1 Ensure the efficient and effective system for referral is maintained and developed.
1.2 Ensure comprehensive holistic assessment of patients for complementary therapies treatment, and evaluation of interventions.
1.3 Provide hands-on complementary therapies.
1.4 Contribute to the development and implementation of effective mechanisms for communicating information concerning patient care including the completion of accurate and comprehensive written records.
1.5 Prioritise and co-ordinate workload of complementary therapies team according to the needs of patients/carers and skills of therapists.
1.6 Provide clinical supervision to complementary therapies team and helpers.
1.7 Advise, support and involve family and carers in providing simple massage following assessment of need.
1.8 Ensure the efficient control, supply and storage of complementary therapy resources, eg oils, tapes, equipment, needles
1.9 Ensure there is an effective system for the supply of clean laundry.
1.10 Comply with the requirements of Professional Code of Conduct and Practice.
1.11 Ensure practice in complementary therapy is evidence-based and encourage the use of research in further development of clinical practice.

#### 2 Management and Development
2.1 Lead the development of policies and procedures for complementary therapies, and participate in the development of the hospice quality assurance programme.
2.2 Manage and develop a team of volunteer

complementary therapists.

2.3 Recruit volunteer complementary therapists in accordance with agreed standards.

2.4 Manage the introduction of other complementary therapies.

2.5 Explore the further development of complementary therapies, eg a service to patients in their homes; the use of essential oils in wound care

2.5.1 Collect and collate statistical data as required by the Hospice Management Team.

2.7 Liaise and collaborate with other complementary therapists in palliative care

3 **Education**

3.1 Educate the multidisciplinary team on the role of available complementary therapies to enable team members to make referrals.

3.2 Participate in staff induction and education programmes.

3.3 Provide support, teaching and advice to clinical staff on complementary therapies.

3.4 Lead and develop the Simple Massage Course for nurses and health care assistants.

3.5 Organise training for volunteers in palliative care and the use of complementary therapies in palliative care

3.6 Be aware of current developments in palliative care and the implications on clinical practice.

4 **General**

4.1 Ensure the welfare and safety of patients, carers, staff and volunteers within the hospice.

4.2 The Hospice expects staff to demonstrate a commitment to their own development, to take advantage of education and training opportunities and develop their professional competence.

4.3 All employees are required to abide by the Health & Safety at Work Act and the Hospice health and safety policies.

4.4 All employees are required to attend a fire lecture annually.

4.5 All employees are required to respect confidentiality applying to all Hospice areas.

4.6 St. Gemma's is a no-smoking area for staff.

4.7 Undertake activities from time to time, representing the Hospice to outside groups or the general public.

This job description is not exhaustive. It will be subject to periodic review and may be amended following discussion between the postholder and employer.

## Appendix G
## Good practice checklist for general volunteers (NCVO 2001)

1. Prior to recruitment, be clear about why you want/need a volunteer;

2. Provide the volunteer with a clear role/task description, identifying anticipated requirement/s of the organisation;

3. Provide the volunteer with an initial induction and training programme;

4. Provide the volunteer with appropriate line management;

5. Add volunteers to organisation charts. Encourage volunteers to participate in the organisation's wider decision-making process;

6. Monitor and acknowledge the contribution that volunteers make to the organisation, to the wider public, to funders and to other volunteers;

7. Ask the volunteer what they seek from their placement and share with the volunteer what you want. Remember that any placement should be by mutual consent;

8. Always offer to reimburse out of pocket expenses. These normally include travel and lunch. Where a placement is away from home, this might also include accommodation and a subsistence allowance;

9. Ensure that health and safety standards are in place and applied equally to all employees (and volunteers). Insurance policies should be extended to cover volunteers;

10. Provide opportunities for volunteers to acquire or develop new or existing skills and assist volunteers who want to gain accreditation towards recognised qualifications;

11. Volunteers should not be recruited to fill the place of paid staff. This could be perceived as exploitation of the volunteer and deprival of someone's livelihood

12. Ensure that the work and contribution of the volunteer adds quality and value to the organisation's aims and objectives;

13. Ensure that Equal Opportunities and/or diversity policies are in place and applied equally to volunteers. Examine the organisation's ways of working for anything that may pose a barrier for some members;

14. Encourage and promote a diverse range of employees at all levels. This will help volunteers from different ethnic groups, ages, disabilities, etc to feel welcome;

15. In order to attract volunteers from groups that the organisation has previously failed to reach, it may be helpful to approach those groups/people directly to establish what would make volunteering with the organisation more appealing to them.

## Appendix H
## Sample role description for volunteer therapist
Used with permission of St. Gemma's Hospice, Leeds

COMPLEMENTARY THERAPIES SERVICE
ROLE DESCRIPTION

Role: Volunteer Complementary
Therapist
Accountable to: Head of Personnel / Volunteers
Responsible to: Complementary Therapies
Co-ordinator

### Overall objective
To provide a service as a member of the Complementary Therapies Team and practice the therapy which has been agreed, in accordance with the policies of St. Gemma's Hospice. The volunteer therapist will also follow the Guidelines for Practice for volunteer therapists.

### Main responsibilities
#### Knowledge
1. Be able to demonstrate a sound understanding of complementary therapies, in particular the therapy for which they are qualified to practice.
2. Be committed to develop skills and knowledge related to the care of patients with active, progressive and advanced disease.

#### Practice
1. Provide a holistic approach to patients and their carers, in collaboration with the other members of the multidisciplinary team, in order to ensure the provision of the highest quality of care.
2. Be competent in therapeutic massage, aromatherapy, reiki or acupuncture
3. Be aware of the patient's diagnoses, treatment, care and current condition.
4. Be aware of contraindications or precautions in relation to the therapy they practice, and be able to adapt a treatment accordingly.
5. Complete the required documentation.
6. Provide feedback, including any adverse effects, to the patient's Team Nurse and the Complementary Therapies Co-ordinator.
7. Participate in 6-8 weekly group clinical supervision with the Complementary Therapies Co-ordinator.
8. Follow the Guidelines for Practice for Volunteers, general and specific to complementary therapies.
9. Follow the Complementary Therapies Policy.

### General
1. Respect the confidentiality of any information held in relation to past or present patients, staff and administration of the hospice.
2. Volunteers are required to abide by (the organisation's) Health & Safety policies.
3. Attend a fire lecture, and moving and handing training annually.
4. (The organisation) is a no-smoking area for staff and volunteers.

May 2002

## Appendix I
# Example of referral form
(Used with permission of St. Gemma's Hospice, Leeds)

## Referral Form for Complementary Therapies
Massage, Aromatherapy, Reiki, Acupuncture

| | |
|---|---|
| Name of referrer: | Date : |
| Designation: | Location/base: |

| | |
|---|---|
| Name of patient | |
| Date of Birth | |
| Next of kin | Significant others: |

| | | |
|---|---|---|
| Inpatient | ☐ Ward: | Date of admission: |
| Day Hospice | ☐ | Attends on: |
| Outpatient | ☐ | Patient's tel. no: |

Priority:     High ☐     Medium ☐     Low ☐

Brief Medical Details

| | |
|---|---|
| Diagnosis | Date: |
| Secondaries | Date: |

| | | | |
|---|---|---|---|
| Recently received/receiving chemotherapy? | YES / NO | When? | Next dose/course due: |
| Recently received/receiving radiotherapy? | YES / NO | When? | Next Rx due: |
| | | Site: | |

Current medication

Other medical diagnosis

Is the patient aware of:

Diagnosis     YES / NO              Prognosis          YES / NO

Any other insight into illness:

Reasons for referral:

| | | | |
|---|---|---|---|
| Anxiety ☐ | Low Mood / Depression ☐ | Diarrhoea ☐ | Constipation ☐ |
| N & V ☐   Pain ☐ | Breathlessness ☐ | Discomfort ☐ | Support & Well-being ☐ |
| Relaxation ☐   Fatigue ☐ | Stress ☐ | Wound care ☐ | Distressing odours ☐ |
| Problems with: | Sleeping ☐ | Body image ☐ | Coping ☐ |

Main concerns:

## PHYSICAL PROBLEMS

| PAIN | COMMENTS |
|---|---|
| Where? | |
| Specific/non specific | |
| Severity | |

### SKIN

| | | |
|---|---|---|
| Itching | ☐ | |
| Dry | ☐ | |
| Sensitive | ☐ | |
| Bruising | ☐ | |
| Lesions | ☐ | |

### MOBILITY

| | | |
|---|---|---|
| No. to transfer | ☐ | |
| Fractures | ☐ | |
| Falls | ☐ | |

### BREATHING

| | | |
|---|---|---|
| Cough | ☐ | |
| Dyspnoea | ☐ | |
| Asthma | ☐ | |

### NEUROLOGICAL

| | | |
|---|---|---|
| Headaches | ☐ | |
| Dizziness | ☐ | |
| Epilepsy | ☐ | |
| Spinal metastases | ☐ | |

### CIRCULATION — COMMENTS

| | | |
|---|---|---|
| Heart condition | ☐ | |
| Thrombosis/clotting disorders | ☐ | |
| High / Low BP | ☐ | |
| Lymphoedema | ☐ | |
| Oedema | ☐ | |

### ANY

| | | |
|---|---|---|
| Colostomy/ileostomy | ☐ | |
| Prostheses | ☐ | |
| Catheter | ☐ | |
| Drains | ☐ | |
| Dressings | ☐ | |
| Pressure sores/wounds | ☐ | |
| Infections | ☐ | |

| | | |
|---|---|---|
| RECENT SURGERY | ☐ | |
| RECENT INJURIES | ☐ | |
| KNOWN ALLERGIES | ☐ | |

### DIGESTIVE

| | | |
|---|---|---|
| Appetite | ☐ | |
| Weight loss | ☐ | |
| Nausea / vomiting | ☐ | |
| Constipation | ☐ | |
| Diarrhoea | ☐ | |

### OTHER

| | | |
|---|---|---|
| Diabetes | ☐ | |
| Urinary problems | ☐ | |

Patients referred for acupuncture  *(must be completed by Day Hospice Team)*

This patient has been screened for contraindications to acupuncture in palliative care by

Dr                                    Date:

Referrer to sign:

## OTHER USEFUL INFORMATION

Appendix J
# Sample Key Worker Initial Assessment Form (condensed)
Used with permission of the Cavendish Centre, Sheffield

## THE CAVENDISH CENTRE / PATIENT: INITIAL ASSESSMENT

Patient's Name: ................................................ Assessor: ................................................

D.o.B: .............................. , ................................ Date: ................................................

Diagnosis: ......................................................... Stage of illness (code): ........................

HOPES and EXPECTATIONS of coming to the Centre: ........................................................

CURRENT SITUATION: ...................................................................................................

Medical History (summarised): ........................................................................................
..........................................................................................................................................
..........................................................................................................................................

Patient's view of the future: ............................................................................................

Current Drug and other therapies: ..................................................................................

FAMILY / SOCIAL SITUATION including SUPPORT e.g. Day Care, Macmillan Nurse: ..........
CONCERNS: ....................................................................................................................

ASSESSORS SUMMARY: .................................................................................................
..........................................................................................................................................
..........................................................................................................................................

MYCAW COMPLETED? YES ☐    NO ☐        If not, why not? ........................................

THERAPY: ........................................................ THERAPIST: ........................................

Reasons for choices: .......................................................................................................

PERMISSION TO WRITE LETTERS TO:            YES ☐    NO ☐

1) .....................................................................................................................................

2) .....................................................................................................................................

3) .....................................................................................................................................

4) .....................................................................................................................................

5) .....................................................................................................................................

RELAXATION GROUP: .....................................................................................................

Action: .............................................................................................................................

ALSO CONSIDER:          - Relaxation tape

                                        - 'Friendly faces'

                                        - Harold Miller Day Care Unit

INFORMATION LEAFLET GIVEN?                    YES ☐    NO ☐

PATIENT DONATION PACK GIVEN?                  YES ☐    NO ☐

Appendix K
## Sample Key Worker Review Assessment Form (condensed)
Used with permission of the Cavendish Centre, Sheffield

## THE CAVENDISH CENTRE / PATIENT: REVIEW ASSESSMENT

Patient's Name:                                    Assessor:

Date:                                              Therapist:

Therapy received:                                  No. of sessions:

Current situation:

Patient's description of specific effects of therapy and their perception of any changes which have taken place and why:(Use patient's own words if possible)

Expectations* met?

Presenting concern(s)* met?

*As noted at initial assessment.

New Concerns:

What might we have done differently?

Are there any other resources which you would like to see us offer?

Patient Donation pack given?           YES ☐   NO ☐

Assessor's Comments:

Interested in Relaxation Class?        YES ☐   NO ☐
Action:
Permission to write?                   YES ☐   NO ☐
Letters to:

Further therapy privately?             YES ☐   NO ☐   POSSIBLY ☐
MYCAW completed?                       YES ☐   NO ☐
If not why not?

# Example of Treatment Record (condensed)
Used with permission of St. Gemma's Hospice, Leeds

## COMPLEMENTARY THERAPIES RECORD
(for the touch therapies)

Name

Date:                                        Therapist:

Review before Treatment

Oils used (if any)

Treatment and observations during treatment

Review after Treatment

Date:                                        Therapist:

Review before Treatment

Oils used (if any)

Treatment and observations during treatment

Review after Treatment

Appendix L (ii )
## Example of Massage Treatment Record (condensed)
Used with permission of The Royal Marsden Hospital

## The Royal Marsden Hospital: Therapeutic Massage Assessment/Treatment Form

| Name | | Hospital No. | | NHS | PP | OP |
|---|---|---|---|---|---|---|
| | | | | DC | IP | |

Ward:

Address · Consultant

· DoB (age)

Tel No

Referral received · Referred by
Reason for referral · Date of first contact
Diagnosis

Medical Information
Surgery
Chemotherapy
Radiotherapy
Other
Allergies

Social History
Problem list
Treatment plan

Referral to other members of the MDT
Therapist's name: · Therapist's signature:

Name: · Hospital No:

| Date | Treatment No | OP  DC  IP  Ward: | Duration | Music |
|---|---|---|---|---|
| Base oil | Essential oils | No drops | Treatment given / positioning | |

Therapist's signature:

| Date | Treatment No | OP  DC  IP  Ward: | Duration | Music |
|---|---|---|---|---|
| Base oil | Essential oils | No drops | Treatment given / positioning | |

Therapist's signature:

## Appendix M
## Participants at the three symposia

| | |
|---|---|
| Judy Abbott | Service User, Sheffield |
| Dr Julian Abel | Weston Hospicecare, Weston-super-Mare |
| Angela Avis MBE | RCN Complementary Therapies Forum |
| Jane Bailey | Salisbury Hospice |
| Jill Bailey | Trafford MacMillan Centre |
| Elizabeth Baines | CancerCare Dorset |
| Ann Barnes | Arthur Rank House, Cambridge |
| Marlene Barry | Springhill Hospice, Rochdale |
| Maggie Brain | Hospice in the Weald, Tunbridge Wells |
| Veronica Bratt | The Primrose Hospice and Cancer Help Centre, Bromsgrove |
| Jeremy Browne | Service User, Hampshire |
| Nadia Brydon | The Haven Trust, London |
| Stella Carmichael | Newcastle Health Action Zone |
| Angela Chisholm | Arthur Rank House, Cambridge |
| Ann Carter | St. Ann's Hospice, Manchester |
| Helen Cooke | Bristol Cancer Help Centre |
| Anna Craven | Service User, North Yorkshire |
| Sara Crisell | Service User, Essex |
| Peter Cross | Service User, Cumbria |
| Lilibet Czyzewska | Service User, Bradford |
| Dr Rosy Daniel | Healthy Bristol |
| Tricia Darnell | The Prince of Wales's Foundation for Integrated Health |
| Beverley de Valois | North Middlesex University Hospital NHS Trust |
| Tony Dougan | Cancer Care (North Lancs and South Lakes) |
| Diana Dunrossil | The Prince of Wales's Foundation for Integrated Health |
| Norman Dunsby | Willowbrook Hospice, Prescot |
| Jeannie Dyer | Royal Marsden Hospital, London |
| Carole Farah | Service User, Swansea |
| Gwyn Featonby | Butterwick Hospice Care, Stockton-on-Tees |
| Frances Fewell | Anglia Polytechnic University |
| Pauline Galloway | Teeside Hospice Care Foundation |
| Terry Gentry | Service User, Middlesbrough |
| Tina Glynn | St. George's Healthcare NHS Trust, London |
| Roma Grant | National Council for Hospice and Specialist Palliative Care Services |
| Russell Hart-Davies | South Leeds PCT |
| Betty Heslop | Service User, Northumberland |
| Dione Hills | The Prince of Wales's Foundation for Integrated Health |
| Sally Hughes | The Prince of Wales's Foundation for Integrated Health |
| Pat Hunter | The Peace Hospice, Watford |
| Sandra Hurd | University Hospital of Leicester NHS Trust |
| Pamela Jack | The Prince of Wales's Foundation for Integrated Health |
| Val Jarvis | Beechwood Cancer Care Centre, Stockport |
| Richard Kane | North Devon Hospice |

| | |
|---|---|
| Dr Jenny Kitchen | The Shropshire and Mid Wales Hospice |
| Dorothy Lambeth | Robert Ogden MacMillan Centre, Leeds |
| Dr Richard Lamerton | Hospice of the Valleys, Tredegar |
| Wendy Leach | Mount Edgcumbe Hospice, Cornwall |
| Dr. Graham Leng | Hospice of the Good Shepherd, Chester |
| Gina Long | South Leeds PCT |
| Karen Loxton | Richard Dimbleby Cancer Information & Support Service, London |
| Peter Mackereth | Christie Hospital NHS Trust, Manchester |
| Dr. Andrew Manasse | The Cavendish Centre for Cancer Care, Sheffield |
| Patricia McDermott | Edenhall Marie Curie Centre, London |
| Deirdre McGuigan | Bristol Children's Hospital |
| Louise Meadan | Marie Curie Centre Holme Tower, Vale of Glamorgan |
| Dr. Alison Morrison | Ardgowan Hospice, Scotland |
| Libby Mytton | The Primrose Hospice and Cancer Help Centre, Bromsgrove |
| Kate Nadkarni | Bradford Cancer Support |
| Gillian Peace | The Cavendish Centre for Cancer Care, Sheffield |
| Lev Pedro | Immune Development Trust, London |
| Margot Pinder | The Prince of Wales's Foundation for Integrated Health |
| Howard Plummer | Sandville Court Self Help Centre, Bridgend |
| Gwyneth Poacher | Sandville Court Self Help Centre, Bridgend |
| Judith Powell | Wakefield Hospice, West Yorkshire |
| Noel Ratcliffe | The Peace Hospice, Watford |
| Dr. Dai Roberts | St. Ann's Hospice, Manchester |
| Robert Ross | Service User, Oxford |
| Serena Scrine | St. Luke's Hospice, Plymouth |
| Sue Smith | Mustard Tree Macmillan Centre, Plymouth |
| Dawn Solomon | Newcastle PCT |
| Dr Dingle Spence | St. Peter's Hospice, Bristol |
| Jacqui Stringer | Christie Hospital NHS Trust, Manchester |
| Jackie Syrett | Dove House Hospice, Hull |
| David Tapper | St. David's Foundation, Newport |
| Elizabeth Taylor | Holistic Resources, Lancashire |
| Gillian Thomas | Edenhall Marie Curie Centre, London |
| Dr Elizabeth Thompson | Bristol Homeopathic Hospital |
| Dr. Elizabeth Thompson | St. Margaret's Somerset Hospice |
| Anna Thomson | The Prince of Wales's Foundation for Integrated Health |
| Chris Walker | Service User, Northumberland |
| Mina West | Cherry Lodge Cancer Care, Barnet |
| Dr Susie Wilkinson | Marie Curie Palliative Care R&D Unit, Royal Free University College Hospital, London |
| Jane Wilkinson | School of Integrated Health Care, University of Westminster |
| Lorraine Williams | The Prince of Wales's Foundation for Integrated Health |
| Maureen Williams | Nursing and Midwifery Council |
| Andrew Wilson | Marie Curie Centre Holme Tower, Vale of Glamorgan |
| Catherine Wood | Dove House Hospice, Hull |
| Yvonne Young | Service User, Swansea |

## Appendix N
# Wider consultative group

| | |
|---|---|
| Lucy Bell | Charing Cross and Hammersmith Hospitals |
| Jo Bray | H.O.P.E. |
| Gordon Brown | Department of Health |
| Anne Cawthorn | University of Manchester |
| Val Chiesa | The Peace Hospice |
| Prof. S.J. Closs | University of Leeds |
| Prof. Jessica Corner | University of Southampton |
| Dr. Michael Dixon | NHS Alliance |
| Dr. Peter Fisher | Royal London Homeopathic Hospital |
| Helen Frances | St. Luke's Hospice, Plymouth |
| Sharon Haffenden | MS Society |
| Sue Hawkett | Department of Health |
| Prof. Irene Higginson | King's College London |
| Caroline Hoffman | Royal Marsden Hospital |
| Wendy Hoy | Macmillan Butterfly Centre, Epsom |
| Dr. Sosie Kassab | Royal London Homeopathic Hospital |
| Steve Kirk | St. Gemma's Hospice, Leeds |
| Gillian Leng | NICE |
| Rosemary Lucey | The Lynda Jackson Macmillan Centre |
| Jo Luthert | Supportive & Palliative Care Guidance |
| Dr. David McGavin | Blackthorn Medical Centre and Trust |
| Heidi MacLeod | MND Association |
| Lynne Morrison | Cancerlink |
| Dr. Charlotte Paterson | Warwick House Medical Centre |
| Helen Press | Sue Ryder Care |
| Prof. Alison Richardson | King's College London |
| Diane Robinson | St. Catherine's Hospice, Scarborough |
| Sheila Scott | Parkinson's Disease Society |
| Dr. Maire Shelly | South Manchester University Hospitals NHS Trust |
| Peter Smith | National Association of Primary Care |
| Elaine Stevens | RCN Palliative Nursing Group |
| Margaret Stevenson | Scottish Partnership Agency |
| Peter Tebbit | National Council for Hospice and Specialist Palliative Care Services |
| Pat Turton | Bristol Cancer Help Centre |
| Debbie Veel | St. Michael's Hospice, Basingstoke |

Aromatherapy Regulatory Working Group
Reflexology Forum
General Council for Massage Therapy
Council of Organisations Registering Homeopaths
The Faculty of Homoeopathy
Acupuncture Association of Chartered Physiotherapists
British Medical Acupuncture Society
British Academy of Western Acupuncture
British Acupuncture Council
British Society of Medical and Dental Hypnosis
UK Confederation of Hypnotherapy Organisations
UK Reiki Federation
British Association of Therapeutic Touch
UK Healers

Appendix O
## Experts consulted

| | |
|---|---|
| Dr. Julian Abel | Weston Hospicecare |
| Rosie Anderson | UK Reiki Federation |
| Eileen Aspinall | St. Gemma's Hospice, Leeds |
| Jill Bailey | ACPOPC |
| Lucy Bell | Charing Cross Hospital |
| Maggie Brain | Hospice in the Weald, Tunbridge Wells |
| Angie Buxton | University College Hospital, London |
| Ann Carter | St. Ann's Hospice, Manchester |
| Elaine Charlesworth | University College Hospital, London |
| Dr. Raj Chopra | Christie Hospital NHS Trust |
| Sara Crisell | Service User |
| Peter Cross | Service User |
| Jeannie Dyer | Royal Marsden Hospital |
| Dr. Jacqueline Filshie | Royal Marsden Hospital |
| David Franchi-Christopher | General Medical Council |
| Stephen Gordon | Society of Homeopaths |
| Prof. John Gruzelier | Imperial College London University |
| Sharon Haffenden | MS Society |
| Annie Hallett | Ipswich Hospital NHS Trust |
| Sarah Hart | Royal Marsden Hospital |
| Liz Hawkins | Univ. of Westminster; Harley Street Clinic |
| Betty Heslop | Northumberland Cancer Support Group |
| Val Hopwood | Acupuncture Assoc. of Chartered Physiotherapists |
| Dr. Sosie Kassab | Royal London Homeopathic Hospital |
| Dr. Jenny Kitchen | St. Peter's Hospice, Bristol |
| Dr. Michelle Kohn | Macmillan Cancer Relief |
| Lyn Lamont | Northern Ireland Cancer Centre, Belfast |
| Dr. Graham Leng | Hospice of the Good Shepherd, Chester |
| Prof. Malcolm McIlmurray | Royal Lancaster Infirmary |
| Peter Mackereth | Christie Hospital NHS Trust, Manchester |
| Dr. Hugh MacPherson | Northern College of Acupuncture |
| Dr. Andrew Manasse | The Cavendish Centre for Cancer Care |
| Gill McCall | St. Thomas' Hospital |
| Dr. McIllmurray | Royal Lancaster Infirmary |
| Heidi MacLeod | MND Association |
| Dr. David Oakley | University College Hospital |
| Jacky Owens | University College Hospital |
| Brenda Peace | UK Healers |
| Jean Sayre-Adams | Sacred Space Foundation |
| Sheila Scott | Parkinson's Disease Society |
| Serena Scrine | St. Luke's Hospice, Plymouth |
| Linda Shuttleworth | St. Gemma's Hospice, Leeds |
| David Simons | The Cavendish Centre for Cancer Care |
| Dr. Mike Stockton | St. Gemma's Hospice, Leeds |
| Jacqui Stringer | Christie Hospital NHS Trust, Manchester |
| Peter Tebbit | NCHSPCS |
| Gill Thomas | Trinity Hospice, London |
| Dr. Elizabeth Thompson | Bristol Homeopathic Hospital |
| Prof. Alan Thompson | Nat. Hospital for Neurology & Neurosurgery |
| Celia Tudor-Evans | College of Traditional Acupuncture |
| Prof. Leslie Walker | University of Hull |
| Joyce West | Aromatherapy Organisations Council |
| Frank Westell | General Council for Massage Therapy |
| Dr. Susie Wilkinson | Marie Curie Palliative Care R&D Unit |
| Julia Williams | University College Hospital |
| Maureen Williams | Nursing and Midwifery Council |
| Dr. Ann Williamson | Brtish Society for Medical and Dental Hypnosis |
| Prof. Steve Wright | Sacred Space Foundation |

Reflexology Forum
Aromatherapy Regulatory Working Group
General Council for Massage Therapy
Council of Organisations Registering Homeopaths
British Acupuncture Council
Acupuncture Association of Chartered Physiotherapists
British Academy of Western Acupuncture
British Medical Acupuncture Society
British Society for Medical and Dental Hypnosis
British Association of Therapeutic Touch
UK Reiki Federation
UK Healers

## Appendix P
## Glossary of terms

| | |
|---|---|
| ACPOPC | Association of Chartered Physiotherapists in Oncology and Palliative Care |
| CT | Complementary therapy / therapies |
| Clients | This term is used interchangeably with patients |
| Clinical services/setting/team | This term is used to refer to services provided within a multidisciplinary conventional health care team |
| DoH | Department of Health |
| GMC | General Medical Council |
| HOPE | HIV/AIDS, Oncology and Palliative Care Education, British Association of Occupational Therapists, specialist group |
| NACTHPC | National Association of Complementary Therapists in Hospice and Palliative Care |
| NCHSPCS | National Council for Hospice and Specialist Palliative Care Services www.hospice-spc-council.org.uk |
| NHS | National Health Service |
| NICE | National Institute for Clinical Excellence www.nice.org.uk |
| NMC | Nursing and Midwifery Council |
| Non-clinical services /setting/team | This term is used to refer to services provided in settings without a multidisciplinary conventional healthcare team. |
| Patients | This term is used interchangeably with 'clients' |
| S & PC | Supportive and palliative Care |

## Appendix Q
# Useful resources

1. Palliative care

Association of Chartered Physiotherapists in
Oncology and Palliative Care
Katherine Malhotra, Secretary of Membership
Physiotherapy Department
Royal Marsden Hospital
Fulham Road
London, SW3 6JJ
Email: acpopc@lineone.net
Website: www.acpopc.org.uk

British Heart Foundation
Head Office
14 Fitzhardinge Street
London, W1H 6DH
Tel: 020 7935 0185
Fax: 020 7486 5820
Email: internet@bhf.org.uk
Website: www.bhf.org.uk

British Lung Foundation
Head Office
78 Hatton Garden
London, EC1N 8LD
Tel: 020 7831 5831
Email: info@britishlungfoundation.com
Website: www.britishlungfoundation.org.uk

Help the Hospices
Hospice House
34-44 Britannia Street
London, WC1X 9JG
Tel: 020 7520 8200
Fax: 020 7278 1021
Email: info@helpthehospices.org.uk
Website: www.helpthehospices.org.uk

Macmillan Cancer Relief
89 Albert Embankment
London, SE1 7UQ
Tel: 020 7840 7840
Fax: 020 7840 7841
Email: cancerline@macmillan.org.uk
Website: www.macmillan.org.uk

Marie Curie Cancer Care
Website: www.mariecurie.org.uk
For all general enquiries, please e-mail
info@mariecurie.org.uk or you can write to their head
offices in England, Scotland, Wales and Northern
Ireland:

Marie Curie Cancer Care England
89 Albert Embankment
London, SE1 7TP
Tel: 020 7599 7777

Marie Curie Cancer Care Northern Ireland
60 Knock Road
Belfast, BT5 6LQ
Tel. 028 9088 2060

Marie Curie Cancer Care Scotland
29 Albany Street
Edinburgh, EH1 3QN
Tel. 0131 456 3700

Marie Curie Cancer Care Wales
Raglan Chambers
63 Frogmore Street
Abergavenny,
Monmouthshire NP7 5AN
Tel: 0187 330 3000

National Council for Hospice and Specialist Palliative
Care Services
1st Floor
34-44 Britannia Street
London, WC1X 9JG
Tel: 020 7520 8299
Fax: 020 7520 8298
Website: www.hospice-spc-council.org.uk

Occupational Therapists - HOPE
Chair: Jill Cooper, Head Occupational Therapist,
Royal Marsden Hospital
Lilac Cottage
Plumpton Lane
Plumpton Green
Nr Lewes
East Sussex, BN7 3AH
Tel: 020 7808 2830
Email: Jill.Cooper@rmh.nthames.nhs.uk

Royal College of Nursing, Complementary Therapies
Forum
Chair, Mrs Angela Avis MBE
Lecturer
Oxford Brookes University
School of Health Care
Dorset House
London Road
Oxford, OX3 7PE
Tel: 01865 485291
Email: aavis@brookes.ac.uk

Terrence Higgins Trust
National Office
52-54 Grays Inn Road
London, WC1X 8JU
Tel: 020 7831 0330
Fax: 020 7242 0121
Email: info@tht.org.uk
Website: www.tht.org.uk

2. Complementary therapies

Acupuncture Association of Chartered
Physiotherapists
Secretariat, Vibeke Dawson
Mere Complementary Practice
Castle Street, Mere
Wiltshire, BA12 6JE
Tel: 01747 861151
Fax: 01747 861717
Email: sec@aacp.uk.com
Website: www.aacp.uk.com

Aromatherapy Regulatory Working Party
Geoffrey Lawler
Independent Chair
The Public Affairs Company
21 Otley Road
Leeds, LS6 3AA

Association of Chartered Physiotherapists in Reflex
Therapy
Alison Stain
3 Whichcote Avenue
Meriden, Coventry
West Midlands
CV7 7LR

Association of Chartered Physiotherapists
Interested in Massage
Tessa Campbell
9 Woodfield Drive
Winchester
Hampshire
SO22 5PY

Bowen technique
The Bowen Forum
Website: www.bowen4health.co.uk

Bristol Homeopathic Hospital
Dr. E.A. Thompson
Consultant Homeopathic Physician and
Honorary Senior Lecturer in Palliative Care
Cotham Hill
Bristol BS6 6JU
Tel:  0117 973 1231
Fax: .0117 923 8759
Email:  elizabeth.thompson@ubht.swest.nhs.uk

British Academy of Western Acupuncture
Tel: 0151 343 9168
Fax: 0151 343 9168
Email: info@bawa-acupuncture.org.uk
Website: www.bawa-acupuncture.org.uk

British Acupuncture Council
63 Jeddo Road
London, W12 9HQ
Tel: 020 8735 0400
Email: info@acupuncture.org.uk
Website: www.acupuncture.org.uk

British Association of Therapeutic Touch
c/o David Lewis
3 Union Street
Carmathen
Carms.
SA31 3DE
Tel. 01267 232715
Email: dlewis@clara.co.uk
Website: www.ttouch.org.uk

British Medical Acupuncture Society
The Administrator
12 Marbury House
Higher Whitley
Warrington
Cheshire, WA4 4QW.
Tel: 01925 730727
Fax: 01925 730492,
Email: admin@medical-acupuncture.org.uk
Website: www.medical-acupuncture.co.uk

British Society of Medical and Dental Hypnosis
Mrs Angela Morris
National Office Secretary
28 Dale Park Gardens
Cookridge
Leeds, LS16 7PT
Tel/Fax: 07000 560309
E-mail: nat.office@bsmdh.org
Website: www.bsmdh.org

Council of Organisations Registering Homeopaths
Peter Mitchell
Treasurer
11 Wingle Tye Road
Burgess Hill
West Sussex, RH15 9HR
01273 878777
Email: homeopathy@platform11.org.uk

Craniosacral therapy
The Cranial Forum
Website: www.cranio.org.uk

The Faculty of Homeopathy
15 Clerkenwell Close
London, EC1R 0AA
Tel: 020 7566 7800.
Fax: 020 7566 7815
Website: www.trusthomeopathy.org

General Council for Massage Therapy
46 Millmead Way
Hertford
SG14 3YH
Tel: 01992 537637
Email: admin@gcmt-uk.org
Website: www.gcmt-uk.org

The Prince of Wales's Foundation for Integrated Health
12 Chillingworth Road
London, N7 8QJ
Tel: 020 7619 6146
Fax: 020 7700 8434
Email: info@fihealth.org.uk
Website: www.fihealth.org.uk

Reflexology Forum
PO Box 2367
South Croydon
Surrey, CR2 7ZE
Tel: 0800 037 0130
Email: reflexologyforum@aol.com

Shiatsu
The General Shiatsu Council
Glebe Cottage
Holywell Road
Castle Bytham
Grantham, NG33 4SL
Email: generalshiatsucouncil@hotmail.com

UK Confederation of Hypnotherapy Organisations
Suite 401
302 Regent Street
London, W1R 6HH
Tel/Fax: 0800 952 0560
E-mail: UKCHO@hypnotherapy.demon.co.uk
Website: www.ukcho.org.uk

UK Healers
Chris Denton
Secretary
PO Box 4137
London, W1A 5FE
Tel: 01943 468476
Email: healing@cpdenton.freeserve.co.uk
Website: www.ukhealers.info

UK Reiki Federation
PO Box 1785
Andover, SP11 OWB
Tel: 01264 773774
Email: enquiry@reikifed.co.uk
Website: www.reikifed.co.uk

3. Complementary therapies in supportive and palliative care

Bristol Homeopathic Hospital
Dr. E.A. Thompson
Consultant Homeopathic Physician and
Honorary Senior Lecturer in Palliative Care
Bristol Homeopathic Hospital
Cotham Hill
Bristol BS6 6JU
Tel. 0117 973 1231
Email: elizabeth.thompson@ubht.swest.nhs.uk

Complementary Therapies in Practice (London and south east)
Karen Loxton, Complementary Therapy Co-ordinator
Richard Dimbleby Cancer Information and Support Service
St. Thomas' Hospital
Lambeth Palace Road
London, SE1 7EH
Tel: 020 7928 9292 Extn. 6012
Email: karen.loxton@gstt.sthames.nhs.uk

Hammersmith Hospitals NHS Trust
Lucy Bell, Complementary Therapy Team Leader
Clinic 8, Outpatients Department
1st Floor
Charing Cross Hospital,
Fulham Palace Road
London W6 8RF
Tel. 020 8383 0463
Email: Lbell@hhnt.org

The Cavendish Centre for Cancer Care
27 Wilkinson Street
Sheffield
South Yorkshire S10 2GB
Tel. 0114 278 4600
E mail: enquiries@cavcare.org

Macmillan Cancer Relief
Dr. Michelle Kohn
Complementary Therapies Medical Adviser
Macmillan Cancer Relief
89 Albert Embankment
London SE1 7UQ
E mail: michellekohn@btinternet.com

National Association of Complementary Therapists in Hospice and Palliative Care
Chair, Freda Magee
29 King's Road
Berkhamsted
Herts, HP4 3BH
Tel: 01442 874226
Email: nacthpc@hotmail.com

Royal London Homeopathic Hospital
Dr. Sosie Kassab
Director of Complementary Cancer Services
Royal London Homeopathic Hospital
Greenwell Street
London, W1W 5BP
Email: sosie.kassab@uclh.org

Royal Marsden Hospital
Dr. Jacqueline Filshie
Consultant in Anaesthesia and Pain Management
The Royal Marsden Hospital
Downs Road
Sutton
Surrey, SM2 5PT
Email: jacqueline.filshie@rmh.nthames.nhs.uk

Caroline Hoffman
Nurse Consultant in Cancer Care (Rehabilitation)
The Markus Centre
The Royal Marsden Hospital
Fulham Road
London, SW3 6JJ
Email: caroline.hoffman@rmh.nthames.nhs.uk

Salford University/Christie Hospital NHS Trust
Peter Mackereth
Lecturer/Practitioner
Rehabilitation Centre
Christie Hospital NHS Trust
Wilmslow Road
Withington
Manchester, M20 4BX
Tel. 0161 446 3795
Email: peter.a.mackereth@virgin.net

St. Ann's Hospice
Ann Carter
Complementary Therapy Co-ordinator
Neil Cliffe Cancer Centre
Wythenshawe Hospital
Southmoor Road
Manchester, M23 9LT
Tel. 0161 291 2913
Email: Ann25@btinternet.com

St. Gemma's Hospice
Marianne Tavares
Complementary Therapies Co-ordinator
329 Harrogate Road
Leeds, LS17 6QD
Tel. 0113 218 5567
Email: mariannet@st-gemma.co.uk

## 4. Websites referred to in these guidelines

British Medical Acupuncture Society
www.medical-acupuncture.co.uk

British Society for Medical and Dental Hypnosis
www.bsmdh.org

National Council for Hospice and Specialist Palliative Care Services
www.hospice-spc-council.org.uk

Skills for Health
www.skillsforhealth.org

The Chartered Society of Physiotherapists
www.csp.org.uk

The Prince of Wales's Foundation for Integrated Health
www.fihealth.org.uk

The Royal College of Nursing
www.rcn.org.uk

The Sacred Space Foundation
www.sacredspace.org.uk

The UK Confederation of Hypnotherapy Organisations
www.ukcho.org

UK Reiki Federation
www.reikifed.co.uk

# 20 References

Abbott N C. Healing as a therapy for human disease: a systematic review. *J. Alternative and Complementary Medicine*. 2000; 6(2):159-169.

Abbott N C. Review of D.J. Benor's (2001) book, *Spiritual Healing: Scientific Validation of a Healing Revolution*, 2002.

ACEVO. *Basic Guide to the Management of Volunteers*. Association of Chief Executives of Voluntary Organisations and National Centre for Volunteering, 1998.

Aglietti L, Roila F, Tonato M et al. A pilot study of metoclopramide, dexamethasone, diphenhydramine and acupuncture in women treated with cisplatin. *Cancer Chemother. Pharmacol* 1990; 26(3):239-40.

Ahles, T.A., et al. Massage therapy for patients undergoing autologous bone marrow transplantation. *Journal of Pain & Symptom Management* 1999;18(3):157-63.

Ahmed HE, Craig WF, White PF, Huber P. Percutaneous electrical nerve stimulation (PENS): a complementary therapy for the management of pain secondary to bony metastasis. *Clin.J Pain* 1998;14(4):320-3.

Alimi D, Rubino C. Leandri EP, Brule SF. Analgesic effects of auricular acupuncture for cancer pain. *J of Pain and Symptom Management*. 2000;19(2):81-2.

Anderson J, Walker MB and Walker LG. The Mood Rating Scale: a brief, acceptable, reliable and valid state measure of normal mood. *Psycho Oncology* 2000; (9):359.

Aung S. The Clinical Use of Acupuncture in Oncology: Symptom Control. *Acupuncture in Medicine* May 1994;12(1):37-40.

BAC. *Code of Ethics and Practice for Counselling Skills*. Rugby, British Association for Counselling, 1989.

Baldry PE. *Myofascial Pain and Fibromyalgia Syndromes*. Churchill Livingstone, 2001.

Ballegaard S, Meyer CN, Trojaborg W. Acupuncture in angina pectoris: does acupuncture have a specific effect? *J. of Internal Medicine* 1991; 229(4):357-62.

Balzarini A, Felisi, Martini A, De Conno. Efficacy of homeopathic treatment of skin reactions during radiotherapy for breast cancer: a randomised, double-blind clinical trial. *British Homeopathic Journal*. 2000; 89:8-12.

Barnes J, Resch KL, Ernst E. Homeopathy for postoperative ileus. *Journal of Clinical Gastroenterology* 1997; 25:628-633.

Barraclough J ed. *Integrated Cancer Care: holistic complementary and creative approaches*. Oxford University Press, 2001.

Bejenke CJ. Benefits of early interventions with cancer patients: A clinician's 15 year observations *Hypnos* 2000; 27(2):75-81.

Bell L. *The Integration of Complementary Therapies within Cancer Services: Guild of Health Writers' Award for Good Practice in Integrated Healthcare*. London, Charing Cross Hospital 1999.

Benor D.J. *Spiritual Healing: Scientific Validation of a Healing Revolution*. Vision Publications, Michigan, 2001

Berman B, Ezzo J, Hadhazy V, Swyers JP. Is acupuncture effective in the treatment of fibromyalgia? *Journal of Family Practice* 1999; 48:213-8.

Billhult A, Dahlberg K. A Meaningful Relief From Suffering: Experiences of Massage in Cancer Care. *Cancer Nursing* 2001; 24(3):180-184.

Birch SJ, Felt RL. *Understanding Acupuncture*. Churchill Livingstone, London, 1999.

Bishop Prof V, Butterworth, Prof T eds. *Clinical Supervision: Conference Proceedings*. NHS Executive, 1994.

Blom M, Dawidson I, Angmar-Mansson B. The effect of acupuncture on salivary flow rates in patients with xerostomia. *Oral Surg Oral Med Oral Pathol* 1992;73:293-298.

Blom M et al. Effects on local blood flux of acupuncture stimulation used to treat xerostomia in patients suffering from Sjogren's syndrome. *J.Oral Rehab* 1993;20:541-548

Blom M, Dawidson I, Fernberg JO, Johnson G, Angmar-Mansson B. Acupuncture treatment of patients with radiation-induced xerostomia. *Eur.J. Cancer B Oral Oncol*, 1996; 32B:182-190.

Blom M, Lundberg T. Long-term follow-up of patients treated with acupuncture for xerostomia and the influence of additional treatment. *Oral Dis*, 2000; 6:15-24

BMA. *Complementary Medicine: New Approaches to Good Practice*. British Medical Association, Oxford University Press, 1993.

Boissell JP, Cucherat M et al. *Critical literature review on the effectiveness of homeopathy: overview of data from homeopathic medicine trials.* Homeopathic Medicine Research Group: Report to the European Commission, Brussels, 1996 p195-210.

Botting D. Review of literature on the effectiveness of Reflexology. *Complementary Therapies in Nursing and Midwifery*, Oct 3 1997; (5)123-30.

Bowles N, Young C. An evaluative study of clinical supervision based on Proctor's three function interactive model. *Journal of Advanced Nursing* 1999; 30(4):958-964.

Bowling A. *Measuring Health: a review of quality of life measurement scales*. 2nd edition. Open University Press, Buckingham, 1997.

Bowsher D. Mechanisms of acupuncture. In Filshie J, White A, eds. *Medical Acupuncture: A Western Scientific Approach*: Churchill Livingstone, Edinburgh 1998. p. 69-82.

Boyd C. *Homeopathic Research Trials: the Evidence*. Unpublished project submitted for final year training in classical homeopathy, 2002.

Bredin M. Mastectomy, body image and therapeutic massage: a qualitative study of women's experience. *Journal of Advanced Nursing* 1999; 29(5):1113-1120.

Buckle J. *Clinical Aromatherapy in Nursing*. California Singular Publishing Group Inc.1995.

Burish T G, Carey M P, Redd W H, Krozely M G, Behavioural Relaxation Techniques in Reducing the Distress of Cancer Chemotherapy Patients. *Oncology Nursing Forum* 1983; 10(3)

Butterworth T, Faugier J. eds. *Clinical Supervision and Mentorship in Nursing*. Chapman & Hall, London, 1992.

Byass R. Auditing complementary therapies in palliative care: the experience of the day-care massage service at Mount Edgcumbe Hospice. *Complementary Therapies in Nursing & Midwifery* 1999; 5:51-60.

Byers D.C. *Better Health with Foot Reflexology*. Ingham Publishing, St. Petersburg, 1983.

Calvert R. A new image for the old adage, *Massage* 37 May/June: 4 1992

Campbell A. *Acupuncture in Practice: Beyond Points and Meridians*. Butterworth-Heinemann, 2001.

Cardena E. Hypnosis in the Treatment of Trauma: a promising, but not fully supported, efficacious intervention. *International Journal of Clinical & Experimental Hypnosis* 2000; 48(2): 225-238.

Cayrou S, Dolbeault S. Development of relaxation techniques in oncology. *Oncology (Huntingt)* Aug 1997; 11(8):1179-89, discussion 1189-95.

Chapman C, Norton R, Paterson C. A Descriptive Outcome Study of 291 acupuncture patients. *Euro J. of Oriental Medicine* 2001; 3(5):48-53.

Cheek DB, Le Cron LM. *Clinical Hypnotherapy*. Grune & Stratton, 1968, p3 and p72

Chiang C-Y, Chang C-T, Chu H-L, Yang L-F. Peripheral afferent pathway for acupuncture analgesia. *Sci.Sin*, 1973; 16: 210-7.

Cho ZH, Chung SC, Jones JP, et al. *New findings of the correlation between acupoints and corresponding brain cortices using functional MRI.* Proc Natl Acad Sci USA 95; 2670-73. 1998.

Cho ZH, Lee SH, Hong IK, et al. Further evidence for the correlation between acupuncture stimulation and cortical activation. Proc. *New Directions in the Scientific Exploration of Acupuncture*. University of California, Irvine, 1999.

Chopra D. *Quantum Healing*. Bantam, New York, 1989.

Christie E, Ward A. *Report on NHS practice-based homeopathy project*. Society of Homeopaths, London, 1996.

Cialdella P, Boissel JP et al. Homeopathic specialties as substitutes for benzodiazepines: double-blind vs placebo study. *Therapie*, Jul-Aug 2001; 56(4):397-402.

CIPD. *Recruitment and Selection*: Quick Fact. Chartered Institute of Personnel and Development, London, 2002. www.cipd.co.uk

Clement-Jones V, McLoughlin L, Tomlin S, Besser GM, Rees LH, Wen HL. Increased beta-endorphin but not met-enkephalin levels in human cerebrospinal fluid after acupuncture for recurrent pain. *Lancet* 1980; 2(8201):946-9.

Clinical Standards Advisory Group. *Services for Patients with Pain*. 2000.

Clover A, Last P, Fisher P et al. Complementary therapy: a pilot study of patients, therapies and quality of life. *Complementary Therapies in Medicine* 1995; 3:129-133.

Cooke B, Ernst E. Aromatherapy: a systematic review. *British Journal of General Practice* June 2000; 493-496.

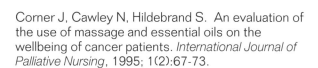

Corner J, Cawley N, Hildebrand S. An evaluation of the use of massage and essential oils on the wellbeing of cancer patients. *International Journal of Palliative Nursing*, 1995; 1(2):67-73.

Coss RS, McGrath P, Caggiano V. Alternative care: patient choices for adjunct therapies within a cancer center. *Cancer Pract* May-June 1998; (3):176-81.

Chartered Society of Physiotherapy. *Physiotherapy and Complementary Medicine*, Information Paper PA48. The Chartered Society of Physiotherapy, London, 2002.

Cucherat M, Boissel JP et al. Evidence of clinical efficacy of homeopathy: a meta-analysis of clinical trials. *European Journal of Clinical Pharmacology* 2000; 56(1):27-33.

Culverwell A, Green D. *An evaluation of cross-disciplinary supervision group for hospice staff*. Unpublished paper, personal communication from D. Green, Leeds University, 1999.

Cumins SM, Brunt AM. Does Acupuncture Influence the Vasomotor Symptoms Experienced by Breast Cancer Patients Taking Tamoxifen? *Acupuncture in Medicine* 2000; 18(1):28.

Cummings M. Teasing Apart the Quality and Validity in Systematic Reviews of Acupuncture. *Acupuncture in Medicine*. 2000;18(2):104-7.

Dantas F, Rampes H. Do homeopathic medicines provoke adverse effects? *British Homeopathic Journal*, 2000; 89(1):S35-38.

De Haes JCJM, Knippenberg FCE, Neijt JP. Measuring psychological and physical distress in cancer patients: structure and application of the Rotterdam Symptom Checklist. *British Journal of Cancer* 1990; 62:1034-8.

Derogatis LR, Morrow GR, Fetting J, Penman D, Piasetsky S, Schmale Am Henrichsm & Carnicke CLM. The prevalence of psychiatric disorder among cancer patients. *Journal of the American Medical Association* 1983; 249:751-757.

Devine EC, Pearcy J. Meta-analysis of the effects of psychoeducational care in adults with chronic obstructive pulmonary disease. *Patient Education and Counselling* 1996; 29(2):167-178.

de Valois B, Clarke E. A retrospective assessment of 3 years of patient audit for an aromatherapy massage service for cancer patients. *The International Journal of Aromatherapy* 2001; 11(3):134-142.

Dibble SL, Chapman J, Mack KA, Shih AS. Acupressure for nausea: results of a pilot study. *Oncology Nursing Forum* Jan-Feb 2000; 27(1):41-7.

Dillon M, Lucas CF. Auricular stud acupuncture in palliative care patients: an initial report. *Palliative Medicine* 1999; 13:253-4.

Dobbs B.Z. Alternative health approaches. *Nursing Mirror* 1985; 160(9);41-42.

Department of Health. *A Vision for the Future: the Nursing, Midwifery and Health Visiting Contribution to Health and Health Care*, Department of Health, London, 1993

Department of Health. *The new NHS: Modern, Dependable*. CM 3807, The Stationery Office, London, 1997

Department of Health. *A First Class Service: quality in the new NHS*, 1998 http://www.open.gov.uk/DOH/public/quality.htm

Department of Health. Clinical Governance: Quality in the new NHS, Leeds, NHS Executive, Department of Health 1999.

Department of Health. *The NHS Cancer Plan: a plan for investment, a plan for reform*. Department of Health, London, Sept 2000.

Department of Health. *Care Standards Act 2000:* effective 1.4.02, Department of Health, London, 2000.

Department of Health. *Guidelines on the Control of Infection in Residential and Nursing Homes*. Public Health Medicine Environmental Group, Department of Health, HMSO, 1996.

Department of Health. *Government Response to the House of Lords Select Committee on Science and Technology's Report on Complementary and Alternative Medicine*. CM 5124. The Stationery Office, London, March 2001.

Donnelly S. Quality-of-life assessment in advanced cancer. *J. Curr Oncol Rep* 2000; Jul 2(4):338-42.

Dorfer L, Moser M, Bahr F, Spindler K, Egarter-Vigl E, Giullen S et al. A medical report from the stone age? *Lancet* 1999; 50:78-80.

Dossey BM et al. *Holistic Nursing* (2nd ed). Aspen Publishers, Gaithersburg, MD, 1995.

Downer SM et al. Pursuit and practice of complementary therapies in cancer patients receiving conventional treatment. *British Medical Journal*, 1994; 309:86-9.

Dundee JW, Ghaly G. Local anesthesia blocks the antiemetic action of P6 acupuncture. *Clin.Pharmacol.Ther*. 1991;50:78-80.

Dundee JW, Ghaly RG, Fitzpatrick KTJ, Lynch GA, Abram WP. Acupuncture to prevent cisplatin-associated vomiting. *Lancet* May 1987; 1083.

Dunn C, Sleep J, & Collett D. Sensing an improvement: an experimental study to evaluate the use of aromatherapy, massage and periods of rest in an intensive care unit. *Journal of Advanced Nursing*, 1995; 21:34-40.

Dunwoody L, Smyth A, Davidson R. Cancer Patient's Experiences and Evaluations of Aromatherapy Massage in Palliative Care. *International Journal of Palliative Nursing* 2002, 8(10):497-504

Duo LJ. Electrical needle therapy for uremic pruritus. *Nephron* 1987;47(3):179-83.

Engretson J, Wardell DW. Biological correlates of Reiki Touch Healing. *Journal of Advanced Nursing*. 2001; 33(4):439-45

Eory A. In vivo skin respiration (CO2) measurements in the acupuncture loci. *Acupunct Electrother Res*, 1984; 9:217-23.

Ernst E, Lee MH. Sympathetic vasomotor changes induced by manual and electrical acupuncture of the Hoku point visualized by thermography. *Pain* 1985; 21(1):25-33.

Ernst E. Complementary AIDS therapies: the good, the bad and the ugly. *International Journal of STD and AIDS* 1997; 8:A1017/1-5.

Ernst E, Pittler MH. The effectiveness of acupuncture in treating acute dental pain; a systematic review. *British Dental Journal*, 1998; 184:443-7.

Ernst E, Rand JI, Stevinson C. Complementary therapies for depression: an overview. *Arch Gen Psychiatry* 1998; Nov; 55(11):1026-32.

Ernst E, White A. Acupuncture for back pain: a meta-analysis of randomized controlled trials. *Arch.Intern.Med*. 1998;158(20):2235-41.

Ernst E. Classical homeopathy versus conventional treatments: a systematic review. *Perfusion* 1999; 12(1):13-15.

Ernst E, Cassileth BR. The prevalence of complementary/alternative medicine in cancer: a systematic review. *Cancer* 1998; 83(4):777.82.

Ernst E, Cassileth BR. How useful are unconventional cancer treatments? *Eur. J. Cancer* Oct 1999; 35(11):1608-13.

Ernst E. Clinical effectiveness of acupuncture; an overview of systematic reviews. In Ernst E, White A, eds. *Acupuncture: a scientific appraisal*. Butterworth-Heinemann, Oxford, 1999. pp.107-27.

Ernst E. Complementary therapies in palliative cancer care. *Cancer* 2001 Jun 1; 91(11):2181-5.

Ernst E. *The Desktop Guide to Complementary and Alternative Medicine*. Harcourt Publishers Ltd, London, 2001.

Evans B. An audit into the effects of aromatherapy massage and the cancer patient in palliative and terminal care. *Complementary Therapies in Medicine* 1995; 3:239-241.

Every R. A Case of Liver Cancer. *The Homeopath* 1999; 74(Summer): 22-25.

Ezzo J, Berman B, Hadhazy VA, Jadad AR, Lao L, Singh BB. Is acupuncture effective for the treatment of chronic pain? A systematic review. *Pain* 2000; 86(3):217-25.

Faithfull S. How many subjects are needed in a research sample in palliative care? *Palliative.Medicine*, 1996;10(3):259-61.

Faugier J, Butterworth T. *Clinical supervision: a position paper*. School of Nursing Studies, University of Manchester, Manchester, 1994.

Fellowes D, Gambles MA, Lockhart-Wood K, Wilkinson SM. *Reflexology for symptom relief in patients with cancer* (Protocol for a Cochrane Review). Cochrane Library, Issue 2. Update Software, Oxford, 2001.

Feng R. Relief of oesophageal carcinomatous obstructuion by acupuncture. *Journal of Traditional Chinese Medicine* 1984; 4:3-4.

Ferrell-Torry A, Glick O. The use of therapeutic massage as a nursing intervention to modify anxiety and the perception of cancer pain. *Cancer Nursing* 1992; 16(20)93-101.

Field TM. Massage therapy effects. *Am.Psychol* 1998; Dec 53(12):1270-81.

Filshie J & Redman D. Acupuncture for malignant pain problems. *European Journal of Surgical Oncology*, 1985;11:389-394

Filshie J. The non-drug treatment of neuralgic and neuropathic pain of malignancy. In Hanks GW, ed. *Pain and Cancer*. Oxford University Press, Oxford, 1988. p.161-93.

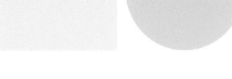

Filshie J. Acupuncture for malignant pain. *Acupuncture in Medicine* 1990; 8(2):38-9.

Filshie J, Penn K, Ashley S, Davis CL. Acupuncture for the relief of cancer-related breathlessness. *Palliative Medicine*, 1996;10:145-150.

Filshie J, Scase A, Ashley S, Hood J. *A study of the acupuncture effects on pain, anxiety and depression in patients with breast cancer* (abstract). Pain Society Meeting, 1997.

Filshie J, White A. The clinical use of, and evidence for, acupuncture in the medical systems. In Filshie J, White A, ed. *Medical acupuncture: A Western Scientific Approach*. Churchill Livingstone, Edinburgh, 1998. p225-94.

Filshie J. Cummings M. Western medical acupuncture. In Ernst E, White A, ed. *Acupuncture: a scientific appraisal*. Butterworth-Heinemann, Oxford, 1999. p.31-59.

Filshie J. Acupuncture in palliative care. *European Journal of Palliative Care*. 2000; 7(2):41-44.

Filshie J, Thompson JW. Acupuncture and TENS. In Simpson KH, Budd K, ed. *Cancer Pain Management: A Comprehensive Approach*. Oxford University Press, Oxford ,2000. pp.188-223

Filshie J. Safety Aspects of Acupuncture in Palliative Care. *Acupuncture in Medicine*. 2001; 19 2):117-122.

Filshie J, Thompson JW. In press, 2002.

Finlay IG, Jones OL. Hypnotherapy in Palliative Care. *Journal of RSM* 1996; 89(9): 493-496

Foundation for Integrated Medicine. *Integrated Healthcare – A Way Forward for the Next Five Years?* Foundation for Integrated Medicine (now The Prince of Wales's Foundation for Integrate Health), London, 1997.

Fisher P. Personal communication, 2003.

Franks A, Ahmedzai S. Current and future research in palliative care. *Palliative Care Today* 1995.

Frei H, Thurneysen A. Homeopathy in acute otitis media in children: treatment effect or spontaneous resolution. *British Homeopathic Journal*, 2001; 90:180-182.

Frei H, Thurneysen A. Treatment for hyperactive children: homeopathy and methylphenidate compared in a family setting. *British Homeopathic Journal*, 2001; 90:183-8.

Friday PJ, Kubal WS. Magnetic resonance imaging: improved patient tolerance using medical hypnosis. *American Journal of Hypnosis*. 1990; 33:80-84.

Gambles M, Crooke M, Wilkinson S. Evaluation of a hospice based reflexology service: a qualitative audit of patient perceptions. *European Journal of Oncology Nursing* 2002; 6(1):37-44.

Garnett M. Sounding it out. *Nursing Times* 1990, Aug 24,90(34)64-67.

General Medical Council. *Duties of a Doctor*. General Medical Council, London, 1998.

General Medical Council. *Standards of Practice*. General Medical Council, London, 1998.

Genuis ML. The use of hypnosis in helping patients control anxiety, pain and emesis: a review of recent empirical studies. *American Journal of Clinical Hypnosis* 1995 Apr; 37(4):316-325

Glasgow Homoeopathic Hospital. *A review of in-patient care integrating complementary and orthodox medicine at Glasgow Homeopathic Hospital*. Interim list report. International Data Collection Centres for Integrative Medicine, 1998.

Gillard Y. Reflexology and radiotherapy. *Footprints* July 1995, 6-17.

Grealish L, Lomasney A, Whiteman B. Foot Massage. *Cancer Nursing* 2000; 23(3): 237-243.

Gordon A, et al. The effects of Therapeutic Touch with patients with osteoarthritis of the knee. *The Journal of Family Practice*, 1998; 47(4):271-277.

Gould AJ, MacPherson H. Patient perspectives on outcomes following treatment with acupuncture. *Journal of Alternative & Complementary Medicine* 2001, 7(3):261-8.

Green *et al.* 1999

Grosz H.J. Hypnotherapy in the management of terminally ill cancer patients. *J Indiana State Med Assoc* 1979 Feb; 72(2):126-9

Guo HF, Tian J, Wang X, Fang y, Hou Y, Han J. Brain substrates activated by electroacupuncture (EA) of different frequencies (II): Role of Fos/Jun proteins in EA-induced transcription of preproenkephalin and preprodynorphin genes. *Brain Res.Mol.Brain Res.* 1996; 43(1-2):167-73.

Hadfield N. The role of aromatherapy massage in reducing anxiety in patients with malignant brain tumours. *International Journal of Palliative Nursing* June 2001; 7(6):279-85.

Hallbert IR, Welander Hansson U, Axelsson K. Satisfaction with nursing care and work during a year of clinical supervision and individualised care: comparison between two wards for the care of severely demented patients. *Journal of Nursing Management* 1994; 1:297-307.

Hallett A. *Unpublished internal audit*. Ipswich Hospital NHS Trust, 1996.

Hallett A. *Unpublished internal audit*. Ipswich Hospital NHS Trust, 2001.

Hammar M, Frisk J, Grimas O, Hook M, Spetz A-C, Wyon Y. Acupuncture Treatment of Vasomotor Symptoms in Men with Prostatic Carcinoma: A Pilot Study. *The Journal of Urology* 1999; 161:853-6.

Han JS, Terenius L, Neurochemical basis of acupuncture analgesia. *Annu.Rev.Pharmacol.Toxicol* 1982; 2:193-220.

Han JS, Chen XH, Sun SL, Xu XJ, Yuan Y, Yan SC et al. Effect of low- and high-frequency TENS on Met-enkephalin-Arg-Phe and dynorphin A immunoreactivity in human lumbar CSF. *Pain* 1991; 47(3);295-8.

Hawkins P, Shohet R. *Supervision in the Helping Professions*. Open University Press, Buckingham, 1989.

He JP, Friedrich M, Ertan AK, Muller K, Schmidt W. Pain-relief and movement improvement by acupuncture after ablation and axillary lymphadenectomy in patients with mammary cancer. *Clinical Exp. Obstet. Gynecology*. 1999; 26(2):81-4.

Health & Safety Commission. *CHIP Part III. Risk phrases*. (Chemical Hazards Information and Packaging) Health and Safety Executive Books, 1994. www.hse.gov.uk/chip/publications.htm

Health & Safety Executive. *COSHH: Safety data sheets for substances and preparations dangerous for supply*. (Control of Substances Hazardous to Health) Health and Safety Executive Books, 1994. www.hse.gov.uk

Health & Safety Executive. *Occupational exposure limits*. Guidance Note EH40 Health and Safety Executive Books, 1994.

National Institutes of Health. *Acupuncture*. NIH Consensus Statement Nov-3-5, 1997;15(5):1-34. http://consensus.nih.gov/cons/107/107_intro.htm

Healthwork UK. *National Occupational Standards for Homeopathy*. Healthwork UK (now Skills for Health), London, 2000.

Healthwork UK. *National Occupational Standards for Aromatherapy*. Healthwork UK (now Skills for Health), London, 2002.

Healthwork UK. *National Occupational Standards for Reflexology*. Healthwork UK (now Skills for Health), London, 2002.

Heap M. *The Psychologist* Nov 1996; 498-501

Heap M, Alden P, Brown RJ, Naish P, Oakley D, Wagstaff G, Walker LG. *The Nature of Hypnosis*. A report prepared by a working party at the request of The Professional Affairs Board of the British Psychological Society, 2001.

Heaven C, Maguire P. *Assessing Patients with Cancer: the content, skills and process of assessment*. Psychological Medicine Group, Christie Hospital NHS Trust, Cancer Research Campaign, Manchester, 1997.

Heidt PR (1981) Effects of Therapeutic Touch on anxiety levels of hospitalised patients. *Nursing Research* 30 (1):32-3.

Hernandez-Reif, M., et al. *Breast cancer patients have improved immune functions following massage therapy*. 2002.

Hills HM, Taylor EE. *Complementary Therapies in Palliative Care: Audit Report* 1.9.00-31.8.01, East Lancashire Integrated Health Care Centre 2001.

Hills HM, Taylor EE. *Complementary Therapies in Palliative Care: Audit Report* 2001-2002. East Lancashire Integrated Health Care Centre 2002.

Hobbs S, Davies P. A critical review of how nurses research massage therapy: are they using the best methods? *Complementary Therapies in Nursing and Midwifery* 1998; 4:35-40.

Hodgson, H. Does reflexology impact on cancer patients' quality of life? *Nursing Standard*, 2000; 14(31):33-8.

Hodkinson E. The Benefits of Reflexology in Palliative Care. *Reflexions*. The Journal of the Association of Reflexologists June 2001; 63:27.

Hodkinson E, Williams J. Enhancing quality of life for people in palliative care settings. *Clinical Reflexology: A Guide for Health Professionals*. Mackereth PA, Tiran D. (ed) Churchill Livingston, London 2002.

Holmes S, Dickerson J. The quality of life design and evaluation of a self-assessment instrument for use with cancer patients. *Int. J. Nurs Stud* 1987; 24(1):5-24.

House of Lords Select Committee on Science and Technology. *Complementary and Alternative Medicine.* HL Paper 123. The Stationery Office, London, November 2000.

Izod D. A patient's perspective. *Complementary Therapies in Nursing and Midwifery.* 1996. 2(3):66-67

Jacknow DS, Tschann JM, Link MP, Boyce WT. Hypnosis in the prevention of chemotherapy-related nausea and vomiting in children: a prospective study. *J Dev Behav Pediatr* 1994 Aug; 15(4):258-64

Jackson AJ. *Massage Therapy.* Optima Books, London, 2000.

Jacobson JS, Workman SB, Kronenberg F. Research on complementary/alternative medicine for patients with breast cancer: a review of the biomedical literature. *Journal of Clinical Oncology,* 2000; Feb; 18(3):668-83.

Jobst K, Chen JH, McPherson J et al. Controlled trial of Acupuncture for disabling breathlessness. *Lancet* 1986; ii:1416-1418.

Johansson K, Lindgren I, Widner H, Wiklund I, Johansson BB. Can sensory stimulation improve the functional outcome in stroke patients? *Neurology* 1993; 43:2189-92.

Johnson MJ, Walker ID, Sproule MW, Conkie J. Abnormal coagulation and deep venous thrombosis in patients with advanced cancer. *Clin.Lab.Haem* 1999; 21, 51-54.

Johnstone PAS, Polston GR, Niemtzow R, Martin PJ. Integration of acupuncture into the oncology clinic. *Palliative Medicine* 2002; 16:235-239.

Jorm AF et al. Effectiveness of complementary and self-help treatments for depression. *Med.J.Aust.* 2002; May 20:176 Suppl:S 84-96.

Joyce M, Richardson R. Reflexology can help MS. *International Journal of Alternative and Complementary Medicine* 1997; 15(7):10-12.

Juhan D. *Jobs Body: a handbook for bodywork.* Station Hill Press, New York, 1987.

Kaptchuk TJ. *Chinese Medicine: The Web that has no Weaver.* Ryder, London, 2000.

Karim K. Conducting research involving palliative patients. *Nursing Standard* Sep27-Oct3 2000; 15(2):34-6.

Kassab S, McCarney R, Van Haselen R, Fisher P. *Homeopathy for Cancer*: A Cochrane Review in planning, 2003.

Keller E. Bzdek UM. Effects of Therapeutic Touch on headache pain. *Nursing Research* 1986; 2 (35):101-105.

King E, Cobbin D, Ryan D. The Reliable Measurement of Radial Pulse: Gender Differences in Pulses Profiles. *Acupuncture in Medicine* 2002; 20(40):160-7.

King E, Cobbin D, Walsh S, Ryan D. Reliable Measurement of Radial Pulse Characteristics. *Acupuncture in Medicine* 2002; 20(40):150-9.

Kirkham S R, Abel J. Placebo-controlled trials in palliative care: the argument against. *Palliative Medicine* 1997;11(6):489-92.

Kirsch I, Montgomery G, Sapirstein G. Hypnosis as an adjunct to cognitive-behavioural psychotherapy, a meta-analysis. *Journal of Consult. Clinical Psychology* 1995; 63:214-220

Kite SM, Maher J et al. Development of an aromatherapy service at a Cancer Centre. *Palliative Medicine* 1998; 12;171-180.

Kleijnen J, Knipschild P, & ter Riet G. Clinical trials of homeopathy. *British Medical Journal,* 1991, Vol 302, Feb 9:316-322.

Kohn M. *Complementary Therapies in Cancer Care*: abridged report of a study produced for Macmillan Cancer Relief, June 1999

Kohn M. Macmillan Directory statistics. In press for publication, 2003

Kotani N, Hashimoto H, Sato Y, Sessler DI, Yoshioka H, Kitayama M et al. Preoperative intradermal acupuncture reduces postoperative pain, nausea and vomiting, analgesic requirement, and sympathoadrenal responses. *Anesthesiology* 2001; 95(2):349-56.

Kraft T. Hypnotherapy for the terminally ill: a review of the first thirty cases. In Heap Med. Hypnotic Contributions; *Proceedings of the Seventh Annual Meeting of the British Society of Experimental and Clinical Hypnosis.* BSECH Publications, Sheffield, 1992

Krieger D. et al. Searching for evidence of physiological change. *American Journal of Nursing* 1979; 79(4):660-663

Lee A, Done ML. The use of nonpharmacologic techniques to prevent postoperative nausea and vomiting: a meta-analysis. *Anesth Analg* 1999; 88:1362-1369.

Leng G. A year of acupuncture in palliative care. *Palliative Medicine* 1999; 13:163-164.

Leslie G. Walker Hypnosis and Cancer: Host Defences, Quality of Life and Survival. *Contemporary Hypnosis*, 1998; 15(1):34-38.

Levitan A A. The use of hypnosis with cancer patients. *Psychiatr Medicine* 1992;10(1):119-31

Lewith G, Kenyon J. Homeopathy. In *Integrated Cancer Care: Holistic, complementary and creative approaches*, ed. J. Barraclough, Oxford University Press, 2001.

Lewith GT, Broomfield J, Prescott P. Complementary Cancer Care in Southampton: a Survey of Staff and Patients. *Complementary Therapies in Medicine*, 2002;10:100-106.

Lewith G, Jonas WB, Walach H. (eds.) *Clinical Research in Complementary Therapies: Principles, Problems and Solutions*. Churchill Livingstone, London, 2002.

Linde K, Melchart D et al. Are the clinical effects of homeopathy placebo effects? A meta-analysis of placebo-controlled trials. *Lancet* 1997; 350:834-43.

Linde K, Melchart D. Randomised Controlled Trials of Individualised Homeopathy: a state-of-the-art review. *The Journal of Alternative and Complementary Medicine* 1998; Vol 4(4):371-388.

Liossi C. White P. Efficacy of clinical hypnosis in the enhancement of quality of life of terminally ill cancer patients. *Contemporary Hypnosis* 2001; 18(3):145-60.

Lockhart-Wood K, Gambles M, Wilkinson S. *Massage and aromatherapy massage for symptom relief in patients with cancer*. Protocol for a Cochrane Review. The Cochrane Library 2001; Issue 2. Update Software, Oxford.

Lynn J. Using complementary therapies: reflexology. *Prof. Nurse* 1996; 11(5):321-2.

Lynn S J, Kirsch I, Barabasz A, Cardena E, Patterson D. Hypnosis as an empirically supported clinical intervention: the state of the evidence and a look to the future. *Int J Clin Exp Hypn*. 2000 Apr;48(2):239-59.

Lu G D, Needham J. *Celestial lancets, a history and rationale of acupuncture and moxa*. Cambridge University Press, Cambridge, 1980.

Lundberg T. Effects of sensory stimulation (acupuncture) on circulatory and immune systems. In:Ernst E, White A, ed. *Acupuncture: a scientific appraisal*: Butterworth-Heinemann, Oxford 1999. pp.93-106.

Ma KW. The roots and development of Chinese Acupuncture: from prehistory to early 20th century. *Acupuncture in Medicine* 1992;10 (supplement); 92-9.

Maa SH, Gauthier D, Turner M. Acupressure as an adjunct to a pulmonary rehabilitation programme. *J.Cardiopulm Rehab* 1997; 17:268-276.

Mackereth P A. Clinical supervision for 'potent' practice. *Complementary Therapies in Nursing and Midwifery* 1997; 3:38-41.

Mackereth P A. An introduction to catharsis and the healing crisis in reflexology. *Complementary Therapies in Nursing and Midwifery* 1999; Jun;5(3):67-74.

Mackereth P A. Clinical Supervision and complementary therapies. *Nurses' handbook of Complementary Therapies* 2nd edition, edited by D. Rankin-Box, Bailiere Tindall, 2001.

Mackereth P A, Tiran D. (eds) *Clinical Reflexology: a Guide for Health Professionals*. Churchill Livingston, London, 2002.

Macmillan Cancer Relief. *Directory of Complementary Therapy Services in UK Cancer Care*. Macmillan Cancer Relief, London, 2002.

MacPherson H, Thomas K J, Walters S, Fitter M. The York acupuncture safety study: prospective survey of 34,000 treatments by traditional acupuncturists. *British Medical Journal* 2001; 323:486-487.

MacPherson H, Thomas K J, Walters S, Fitter M. A Prospective Survey of Adverse Events and Treatment Reactions following 34,000 Consultations with Professional Acupuncturists. *Acupuncture in Medicine* 2001; 19(2):93-102.

Maguire P, Faulkner A, Regnard C. Eliciting the current problems of the patient with cancer – a flow diagram. *Palliative Medicine* 1993; 7:151-6.

Maguire P, Heaven C. *Assessing Patients with Cancer: the content, skills and process of assessment*. Cancer Research Campaign, Psychological Medicine Group, Christie Hospital, Manchester, 1997.

Mallett J, Dougherty L (eds). *Clinical Nursing Procedures*, 5th edition. Royal Marsden Hospital. Blackwell Science Ltd, Oxford, 2000.

Mann F. *Reinventing Acupuncture*. Butterworth Heinemann, 2000.

Manasse A. *The Place of Complementary Therapy in the Care of People with Cancer*. Personal communication, 2001.

Manderson C, Weller R, Wilcock A, Ernst E et al. *Effect of aromatherapy massage on patients attending for day care: a randomised controlled pilot study*. Hayward House Macmillan SPC Unit, Nottingham City Hospital, 2001.

Marchioro G, Azzarello G, Viviani F, Barbato F, Pavanetto M, Rosetti F, Pappagallo GL, Vinante O. *Hypnosis in the treatment of anticipatory nausea and vomiting in patients receiving cancer chemotherapy.* Department of Oncology, Local Health Unit No. 13, Noale, Italy, 2000.

Mayer DJ. Acupuncture: an evidence-based review of the clinical literature. *Annu Rev Med* 2000; 51:49-63.

McMillan CM, Dundee JW, Abram WP. Enhancement of the antiemetic action of the Ondansetron by transcutaneous electrical stimulation of P6 antiemetic points in patients having highly emetic cytotoxic drugs. *British Journal of Cancer* 1991; 64: 971-2.

McNamarra P. *Massage for People with Cancer*. The Cancer Resource Centre, Wandsworth, London, 1999.

Meares A. What can the cancer patient expect from intensive meditation? *Aust Fam Physician* May 1980;9(5):322-5.

Meek SS. Effects of slow stroke back massage on relaxation in hospice clients. *Image* 1993; 25:17-21.

Melchart D, Linde K, Fisher P, White A, Allais G, Vickers A et al. Acupuncture for recurrent headaches: A systematic review of randomised controlled trials. *Cephalalgia* 1999; 19:779-86.

Melzack R, Stillwell DM, Fox EJ. Trigger points and acupuncture points for pain, correlations and implications. *Pain*, 1977; 3:3-23.

Melzack R. Folk Medicine and the Sensory Modulation of Pain. In Melzack R, Wall PD, editors. *Textbook of Pain*. Churchill Livingstone, Edinburgh, 1994. p.1207-17.

Meyer TJ, Mark MM. Effects of psychosocial intervention with adult cancer patients; a meta-analysis of randomised experiments. *Health Psychology* 1995;14:101-108

Micozzi M.S. (ed) *Fundamentals of complementary and alternative medicine*. Churchill Livingston, New York, 1996.

Milligan M, Fanning M, Hunter S, Tadjali M, Stevens E. Reflexology Audit: Patient Satisfaction, Impact on Quality of Life and Availability in Scottish Hospice. *International Journal of Palliative Nursing* 2002, 8(10):489-496.

Montgomery GH, David D, Winkel G, Silverstein JH, Bovbjerg DH. The effectiveness of adjunctive hypnosis with surgical patients: a meta-analysis. *Anesth Analg* Jun 2002; 94(6):1639-45.

Morin CM, Culbert JP, Schwartz SM. Non-pharmacological interventions for insomnia: a meta-analysis of treatment efficacy. *American Journal of Psychiatry*; 1994; 151(8):1172-1180.

Muscari-Tomiaoli Allegri R, Miali E et al. Observational study of quality of life in patients with headache receiving homeopathic treatment. *British Homeopathic Journal* 2001; 90:189-197.

National Council for Hospice and Specialist Palliative Care Services. *Raising the Standard - Clinical Governance for Voluntary Hospices*. National Council for Hospice and Specialist Palliative Care Services, 2000.

National Council for Hospice and Specialist Palliative Care Services. *Definitions of Supportive and Palliative Care – A Consultation Paper*. National Council for Hospice and Specialist Palliative Care Services, June 2002.

National Council for Hospice and Specialist Palliative Care Services. *Turning Theory into Practice - Practical Clinical Governance for Voluntary Hospices*. National Council for Hospice and Specialist Palliative Care Services, 2002(a)

National Council for Voluntary Organisations. *Volunteering: a Code of Good Practice*. London Compact Working Group, Home Office and National Council for Voluntary Organisation, 2001.

National Federation of Spiritual Healers. *What is Spiritual Healing?* Middlesex, National Federation of Spiritual Healers, 1998

National Institute for Clinical Excellence. *Guidance on Cancer Services: Improving Supportive and Palliative Care for Adults with Cancer*. Second consultation document. National Institute for Clinical Excellence, London, September 2002.

Neate T, Neate A. Healing the whole person. *Integrated Cancer Care*. ed. J. Barraclough. Oxford University Press, Oxford, 2001

Nursing and Midwifery Council. *Code of Professional Conduct*. Nursing and Midwifery Council, London, 2002(a).

Nursing and Midwifery Council. *Consent*. Nursing and Midwifery Council, London, 2002(b).

Nursing and Midwifery Council. *Practitioner/Client Relationship*. Nursing and Midwifery Council, London, 2002(c).

Nursing and Midwifery Council. *Confidentiality*. Nursing and Midwifery Council, London, 2002(d).

Nursing and Midwifery Council. *Complementary and alternative therapies*. Nursing and Midwifery Council, London, 2002(e)

Oberbaum M et al. A randomised controlled trial of the homeopathic medication, Traumeel S(R) in the treatment of chemotherapy-induced stomatitis in children undergoing stem cell transplantation. *Cancer* August, 2001.

Oleson T, Flocco W. Randomised controlled study of pre-menstrual symptoms treated with ear, hand and foot reflexology. *Obstetrics and Gynecology* 1993; 82:906-911.

Olsen M. et al. Therapeutic Touch & Post Hurricane Hugo Stress *Journal of Holistic Nursing* 1992; 10 (2):120-136.

Oneschuk D. Complementary therapy use: a survey of community and hospital based patients with advanced cancer. *Palliative Medicine* 2000; 14:432-434.

Owens J. Personal communication. 2002

Pan CX, Morrison RS, Ness J, Fugh-Berman A, Leipzig RM. Complementary and alternative medicine in the management of pain, dyspnoea, and nausea and vomiting near the end of life: a systematic review. *Journal of Pain Symptom Management*, 2000; Nov;20(5):374-87.

Patel M, Gutzwiller F, Paccaud F, Marazzi A. A meta-analysis of acupuncture for chronic pain. *International Journal Epidemiology*, 1989;18(4):900-6.

Paterson C. Measuring outcome in primary care: a patient-generated measure, MYMOP, compared to the SF-36 health survey. *BMJ* 1996; 312:1016-20.

Paterson C, Britten N. In pursuit of patient centred outcomes: a qualitative evaluation of MYMOP, Measure Your Medical Outcome Profile. *Journal of Health Services Research & Policy* 2000; 5:27-36.

Paterson C et al. Measure Your Concerns and Well-Being: outcome measure currently awaiting validation process. 2002.

Peace G, Manasse A. The Cavendish Centre for integrated cancer care: assessment of patients' needs and responses. *Complementary Therapies in Medicine*, 2002; 10: 33-41.

Penson J. Complementary therapies: making a difference in palliative care. *Complementary Therapies in Nursing and Midwifery* 1998; 4:77-81.

Peuker E, Gronemeyer D. Rare But Serious Complications of Acupuncture: Traumatic Lesions. *Acupuncture in Medicine* 2001;19 (2):103-8.

Pomeranz B. Acupuncture Analgesia: Basic Research. In Stux G, Hammerschlag R, editors. *Clinical Acupuncture; Scientific Basis*. Springer-Verlag, Berlin, 2001. pp.1-28.

Poulain P, Pichard Leadri E, Laplanche A, Montange F, Bouzy J, Truffa-Bachi J. Electroacupuncture Analgesia in Major Abdominal and Pelvic Surgery: A Randomised Study. *Acupuncture in Medicine*, 1997; XV(1):10-3.

Preece J. Introducing abdominal massage in palliative care for the relief of constipation. *Complementary Therapies in Nursing and Midwifery*. 2002. 8(2):101-105.

Price H, Lewith G, Williams C. Acupressure as an antiemetic in cancer chemotherapy. *Complementary Medical Research* 1991;5:93-4.

Price S and Price L. *Aromatherapy for Health Professionals*. Churchill Livingstone, London, 1995.

Prince of Wales's Foundation for Integrated Health. Information gathered from 100 guidelines, policies and protocols submitted by palliative care units and teams to the Foundation for Integrated Medicine, (former name of The Prince of Wales's Foundation for Integrated Health), 2001.

Prince of Wales's Foundation for Integrated Health. *Complementary therapies in palliative care: developing national guidelines*. Unpublished reports of three consultative symposia. The Prince of Wales's Foundation for Integrated Health, London, 2002.

Quinn J F. *An investigation into the effect of therapeutic touch done without physical contact on state anxiety of hospitalised cardiovascular patients*. Dissertation Abstracts International 1982; 43: 1797b.

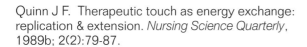

Quinn J F. Therapeutic touch as energy exchange: replication & extension. *Nursing Science Quarterly*, 1989b; 2(2):79-87.

Quinn J F. Holding sacred space, the nurse as a healing environment. *Holistic Nursing practice*, 1992; 6(4):26-35.

Quinn JF. & Strelkaukas A. Psychoimmunologic effects of therapeutic touch on practioners & recently bereaved recipients; a pilot study. *Advanced Nursing Science* 1993; 15(13-26).

Rees R W, Feigel I, Vickers A, Zollman C, McGurk R, Smith C. Prevalence of complementary therapy use by women with breast cancer: a population-based survey. *E. Journal of Cancer* 2000; 36:1359-1364.

Reilly D. *The evidence for homeopathy*. Academic Dept for Homeopathy, Grampian Health Board, Glasgow, 1995.

Research Group of Acupuncture Anaesthesia. Effect of acupuncture on pain threshold of human skin. *China Medical Journal*. 1973; 3:151-7.

Richardson J. *Evidence for Best Practice*. Presented at Annual Conference of Royal College of Nursing Complementary Therapies in Nursing Forum 2001, Oxford (based on Richardson J, Jones C, Pilkington K. Complementary therapies: what is the evidence for their use. Professional Nurse, 2001, 17(2):96-99.

Richardson M A, Ezzo J, Vickers A, Allen C, Lao L, Zhang G, Ramirez G. *Acupoint stimulation for chemotherapy-induced nausea and vomiting*. Presentation at International Scientific Conference on Complementary, Alternative and Integrative Medicine Research, San Francisco May 17-19 2001.

Richardson M A, Allen C, Ezzo J, Lao L, Ramirez G, Ramirez T, Zhang G. *Acupuncture for chemotherapy-induced nausea or vomiting among cancer patients*. (Protocol for a Cochrane review). The Cochrane Library 2001, Issue 2; Update Software, Oxford.

Richter A, Herlitz J, Hjalmarson A. Effect of acupuncture in patients with angina pectoris. *European Heart Journal*, 1991; Feb; 12(2):175-8.

Riley D, Fischer M, Singh B, et al. Homeopathy and conventional medicine: an outcomes study comparing effectiveness in a primary care setting. *Journal of Alternative and Complementary Medicine*, 2001; 7:149-59.

Rogers M E. *An Introduction to the Theoretical Basis of Nursing*. F Davis, Philadelphia, 1970.

Roscoe JA, Morrow GR, Bushunow P, Tian L, Matteson S. Acustimulation Wristbands for the Relief of Chemotherapy-Induced Nausea. *Alternative Therapies* 2002; 8(4):56-63.

Ross CSK, Hamilton J, Macrae G, Docherty C, Gould A, Cornbleet MA. A Pilot Study to Evaluation the Effect of Reflexology on Mood and Symptom Rating of Advanced Cancer Patients. *Palliative Medicine*, 2002, 16(6):544-545

Roth LU, Maret-Maric A, Adler RH, Neuenschwander BE. Acupuncture Points have Subjective (Needling Sensation) and Objective (Serum Cortisol Increase) Specificity. *Acupuncture in Medicine*, 1997;15(1):2-5.

Royal College of Nursing. *Complementary therapies: a consumer checklist*. Royal College of Nursing, London, 1993.

Royal London Homoeopathic Hospital. *The Evidence Base of Complementary Medicine*. 2nd ed. The Royal London Homoeopathic Hospital, London, 1999.

Russell JK. Bodywork: The Art of Touch. *Nurse Practitioner Forum* 1994; Vol.5 No.2 (June)85-90.

Rydholm M, Strang, P. Acupuncture for patients in hospital-based home care suffering from xerostomia. *Journal of Palliative Care* 1999;15(4):20-3.

Sackett DL, Rosenberg WMC, Gray JAM, Haynes RB, Richardson WS. Evidence based medicine: what it is and what it isn't. *BMJ* Jan 1996. (312):71-72.

Sayre Adams J. Wright S. *Therapeutic Touch*. Churchill Livingstone, London, 2001.

Schoenberger NE. Research on hypnosis as an adjunct to cognitive-behavioral psychotherapy. *International Journal of Clinical & Experimental Hypnosis* April 2000; 48(2):154-69.

Scrine S. Personal communication. 2002.

Shaly JC, Chaloner K, Max MB et al. Acupuncture and Amitrptylline for pain due to HIV-related neuropathy: a randomised controlled trial. *JAMA* 1998; 280:1590-1595.

Shang C. The past, present and future of meridian system research. *Clinical Acupuncture: Scientific Basis* eds Stux G & Hammerschlag R. Springer, 2001.

Sharples F, Van Haselen R. *Patients' perspective on using a complementary medicine approach to their health : survey*. Royal London Homeopathic Hospital, London, 1998.

Shen J. Wenger N, Glaspy J, Hays RD, Albert PS, Choi C et al. Electroacupuncture for control of myeloablative chemotherapy-induced emesis: A randomized controlled trial. *JAMA* 2000; 284(21):2755-61.

Sims, S. Slow stroke back massage for cancer patients. *Nursing Times* 1986; 82(47):47-50.

Sindhu F. Are non-pharmacological nursing interventions for the management of pain effective: a meta-analysis. *J. of Advanced Nursing*; 1996; 24:1152-1159.

Sjolund B, Terenius L, Eriksson M. Increased cerebrospinal fluid levels of endorphins after electro-acupuncture. *Acta Physiol Scand*. 1977;100(30):382-4.

Sloman R. Relaxation and imagery for anxiety and depression control in community patients with advanced cancer. *Cancer Nurs*. 2002 Dec; 25(6):432-5.

Smith FF. *Inner Bridges, a guide to energy movement and body structure*. Humanics, Atlanta, Georgia, 1990. pp.78-79.

Smith LA, Oldman AD, McQuay HJ, Moore RA. Teasing apart quality and validity in systematic reviews: an example from acupuncture trials in chronic neck and back pain. *Pain*, 2000; 83(1-2):119-32.

Smith MC, Holcombe JK, Stullenbarger E. A meta-analysis of intervention effectiveness for symptom management in oncology nursing research. *Oncology Nursing Forum* 1994; 21(7):1201-10.

Spene D. *Clinical outcome audit, Bristol Homeopathic Hospital*. Conference Proceedings: Improving the Success of Homeopathy 2, Royal London Homoeopathic Hospital, London, 1999. p.75.

Spiegel D, Bloom JR. Group therapy and hypnosis reduce metastatic breast carcinoma pain. *Psychosom Med* Aug 1983; 45(4):333-9.

Spiegel D, Hunt T, Dondershine HE. Dissociation and hypnotisability in post traumatic stress disorder. *American Journal of Psychiatry* 1988; 145:301-305.

Spiegel D. Facilitating emotional coping during treatment. *Cancer* 1990 Sep 15; 66 (6 Suppl):1422-6.

Spiegel D. Moore R. Imagery and hypnosis in the treatment of cancer patients. *Oncology (Huntington)* Aug 1997; 11(8):1179-89.

Spielberger CD et al. *Manual for the State-Trait Anxiety* Inventory Palo Alto, Calif, Counselling Psychologists Press, 1983.

Spira JL, Spiegel D. Hypnosis and related techniques in pain management. *Hospice Journal* 1992; 8 (1-2): 89-119.

Stanley RO, Rose L, Burrows GD. Professional training in the practice of hypnosis: the Australian experience. *Am.J.Clin.Hypn*. July 1998; 41(1):29-37

Stannard D. Pressure prevents nausea. *Nursing Times*. 1989; 85:33-4.

Steggles S. The use of cognitive-behavioral treatment including hypnosis for claustrophobia in cancer patients. *American Journal of Clinical Hypnosis* April 1999; 41(4):319-26.

Stephenson C. Complementary therapies in cancer care: an NHS approach. *Intl Journal of palliative Nursing* 1996; 2.1.15-18.

Stephenson, N. *The effects of foot reflexology on anxiety and pain in patients with breast and lung cancer*. University of South Carolina, 1997. p. 134.

Stephenson, N .L., Weinrich, S.P. and Tavakoli, A.S. The effects of foot reflexology on anxiety and pain in patients with breast and lung cancer. *Oncology Nursing Forum*, 2000; 27(1):67-72.

Stetter F, Kupper S. Autogenic training: a meta-analysis of clinical outcome studies. *Appl Psychophysiol Biofeedback* March 2002; 27(1):45-98.

Stone J. *An Ethical Framework for Complementary and Alternative Therapies*. London, Routledge, 2002.

Syrjala KL, Donaldson GW, Davis MW, Kippes ME, Carr JE. Relaxation and imagery and cognitive-behavioral training reduce pain during cancer treatment: a controlled clinical trial. *Pain* November 1995; 63(2):189-98.

Talal N et al. The clinical effects of electrostimulation on salivary function of Sjogrens syndrome patients:a placebo controlled study. *Rheumatol Int* 1992; 12:43-45.

Tanner R. *Reflexology Policy Document: Improving Quality of Life in Palliative Care*. Personal communication. 2000.

Taylor E. Personal communication 2002.

ter Riet G, Kleijnen J, Knipschild P. Acupuncture and chronic pain: a criteria-based meta-analysis. *Journal of Clinical Epidemiology* 1990; 43(11);1191-9.

Thomas KJ, Fall M, Nicholl J. Access to complementary medicine via general practice. *British Journal of General Practice* 2001; 51(462):25-30.

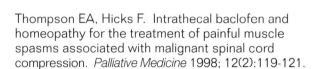

Thompson EA, Hicks F. Intrathecal baclofen and homeopathy for the treatment of painful muscle spasms associated with malignant spinal cord compression. *Palliative Medicine* 1998; 12(2):119-121.

Thompson EA. Using homeopathy to offer supportive cancer care, in a National Health Service outpatient setting. *Complementary Therapies in Nursing & Midwifery* April 1999; 5(2):37-41.

Thompson EA. Personal communication from Dr. Elizabeth Thompson, Consultant, Bristol Homeopathic Hospital, 2002.

Thompson EA, Reilly D. The homeopathic approach to symptom control in the cancer patient: a prospective observational study. *Palliative Medicine* May 2002(a); 16(3):227-33.

Thompson EA, Douglas E, Norrie, Reilly. *A pilot randomised placebo-controlled trial of homeopathy in the management of menopausal symptoms in breast cancer survivors.* Personal communication from author, awaiting submission for publication. 2002(b).

Thompson EA, Reilly D. *The homeopathic approach to the treatment of symptoms of oestrogen withdrawal in the breast cancer patient. A prospective observational study.* Personal communication from author, awaiting publication. 2002(b).

Thompson JW, Filshie J. Transcutaneous electrical nerve stimulation and acupuncture. In Doyle D, Hanks GWC, MacDonald M eds. *Oxford textbook of palliative medicine*, 2nd ed. Oxford University Press, Oxford, 1998. pp. 421-37.

Tougas G, Yuan LY, Radamaker JW, Chiverton SG, Hunt RH. Effect of acupuncture on gastric acid secretion in healthy male volunteers. *Digestive Diseases and Sciences*, 1992; 37(10):1576-82.

Tingle J. Clinical supervision is an effective risk management tool. *British Journal of Nursing* 1995; 4(14)794-795.

Tiran D. Reviewing theories and origins. *Clinical Reflexology: Guide for Health Professionals.* Mackereth P.A. & Tiran D. (eds) Churchill Livingston, London, 2002.

Tisserand R. *Aromatherapy for Everyone*. Penguin, London, 1988.

Tisserand R, Balacs T. *Essential Oil Safety*. Churchill Livingstone, London, 1995.

Towlerton G, Filshie J, O'Brien M, Duncan A. Acupuncture in The control of vasomotor symptoms caused by tamoxifen. *Palliative Medicine* 1999; 13(5):445.

Trijsburg RW, van Knippenberg FC, Rijpma SE. Effects of psychological treatment on cancer patients: a critical review. *Psychosomatic Medicine* Jul-Aug 1992; 54(4):489-517.

Trousdell P. Reflexology meets emotional needs. *International Journal of Alternative and Complementary Medicine* November 1996; 9-13

Ulvnas-Moberg K, Bruzelius G, Alster P, Lundeberg T. The antinociceptive effect of non-noxious sensory stimulation is mediated partly through oxytocinergic mechanisms. *Acta Physiol Scand* 1993; 149(20):199-204.

Van der Riet. Massaged embodiment of cancer patients. *Aust.J.Holist.Nursing* April 1999; 6(1):4-13.

Van Tulder MW, Ostelo RW, Vlaeyen JW, Linton SJ, Morley SJ, Assendelft WJ. Behavioural treatment for chronic low back pain. *Cochrane Database.Syst.Rev*, 2000; (2):CD002014.

Vanessa C. Johnson, Leslie G. Walker, Steven D. Heys, Paul H. Whiting and Oleg Eremin. Can relaxation training and hypnotherapy modify the immune response to stress, and is hypnotizability relevant? *Contemporary Hypnosis* 1996; 13(2):100-l08.

Vickers A & Zollman C. ABC of complementary medicine: Acupuncture. British Medical Journal 1999; 9 Oct; 319:973-976.

Vickers AJ. Can acupuncture have specific effects on health: a systematic review of acupuncture antiemesis trials. *Journal of the Royal Society of Medicine* 1996; 89:303-311.

Vincent C. Principles of risk and safety. *Acta Neurochir.Suppl* 2001;78:3-11.

Vincent CA. Acupuncture research: why do it? *Complementary Medical Research* 1992; 6(1):21-4.

Voluntary Sector National Training Organisation. *National Occupational Standards for Managing Volunteers: Functional Map of Managing Volunteers,* Draft 2. Voluntary Sector National Training Organisation, London, 2002.

Vozianov AF, Simeonova NK. Homeopathic treatment of patients with adenomas of the prostate. *British Homeopathic Journal*, 1990; 79:148-151.

Walker L.G., Dawson A.A., Pollet S.M., Ratcliffe M., and Hamiton L. Hypnotherapy for Chemotherapy Side Effects. *British Journal of Experimental and Clinical Hypnosis* 1988; 5(Z):79-82

Walker LG et al. Hypnotherapy for Chemotherapy Side Effects. *British Journal of Experimental and Clinical Hypnosis* 1988;5(2):79-82

Walker LG, Lolley J, Dawson AA, Ratcliffe MA. Hypnotherapy for chemotherapy side effects – further developments. in M.Heap ed. *Hypnotic Contributions, Proceedings, Seventh Annual Conference*. British Society of Experimental and Clinical Hypnosis, BSECH Publications, Sheffield. pp 63-71.

Walker LG. Hypnosis with Cancer Patients. American *Journal of Preventive Psychiatry and Neurology*. 1992, Fall;3:3

Walker LG, Eremin O. Psychoneuroimmunology: a new fad or the fifth therapeutic modality? *American Journal of Surgery* 1995; 170:2-4

Walker LG. Hypnosis and Cancer: Host Defenses, Quality of Life and Survival. *Contemporary Hypnosis* 1998;15(1):34-38

Walker LG, Walker MB, Ogston K, Heys SD, Ah-See AK, Miller ID, Hutcheon AW, Sarkar TK, Eremin O. The psychological, clinical and pathological effects of relaxation training and guided imagery during primary chemotherapy. *British Journal of Cancer* April 1999; 80(1-2):262-8.

Ward A. *Pilot project report on NHS practice-based homeopathy*. Society of Homeopaths, London, 1994.

Watson M and Greer S. Development of a questionnaire measure of emotional control. *Journal of Psychosomatic Research* 1983, 27, 299-305.

Weinrich SP, Weinrich MC. The effect of massage on pain in cancer patients. *Applied Nursing Research* 1990; 3:140-145.

Weiss SJ. The language of touch. *Nursing Research* 1979; 28(2)76-80.

Wen HL. Cancer pain treated with acupuncture and electrical stimulation. *Mod.Med.Asia* 1977; 13(2):12-6.

Westcombe AM, Gambles MA, Young T, Love SB, Lucey RA, Barnes K, Cubbin S, Fellowes D, Ramirez AJ, Maher EJ, Wilkinson SM. Learning the hard way! Setting up an RCT of aromatherapy massage for patients with cancer. *Palliative Medicine*. (In press.)

Westland G. Massage as a Therapeutic Tool. *Journal of Occupational Therapy* April 1993; 56(4):129-134 and May 56(5):177-180.

White A. Neurophysiology of acupuncture analgesia. In Ernst E, White, eds. *Acupuncture : A Scientific Appraisal*. Butterworth-Heinemann, Oxford, 1999. pp. 60-92.

White A. Acupuncture research methodology. In Lewith G, Jonas WB, Walach H. eds. *Clinical Research in Complementary Therapies*. Churchill Livingstone, Edinburgh, 2002.

White A, Hayhoe S, Hart A, Ernst E. Survey of Adverse Events Following Acupuncture (SAFA): a Prospective Study of 32,000 Consultations. *Acupuncture in Medicine* 2001; 19(20):84-92.

White AR, Filshie J, Cummings TM. Clinical trials of acupuncture: consensus recommendations for optimal treatment, sham controls and blinding. *Complementary Therapies in Medicine*, 2001; 9(4):237-45.

White P. Complementary medicine treatment of cancer; a survey of provision. *Complementary Therapy Medicine*, 1998; 6:10-13.

World Health Organisation. *Cancer Pain Relief and Palliative Care*. Technical report series 804. World Health Organisation, Geneva, 1990 – update April 2002.

Wilkes E. *Complementary Therapy in Hospice and Palliative Care*. SheffieldTrent Palliative Care Centre and Help the Hospices, 1992.

Wilkie, D.J., et al. Effects of massage on pain intensity, analgesics and quality of life in patients with cancer pain: a pilot study of a randomized clinical trial conducted within hospice care delivery. *Hospice Journal - Physical, Psychosocial, & Pastoral Care of the Dying*, 2000; 15(3):31-53.

Wilkinson, S., Aromatherapy and massage in palliative care. *International Journal of Palliative Nursing*, 1995; 1(1):21-30.

Wilkinson, S., et al. An evaluation of aromatherapy massage in palliative care. *Palliative Medicine*, 1999; 13(5):409-17.

Wilkinson S, Ramirez A, Maher J, Sun Myint et al. *A randomised controlled trial to evaluate the use of aromatherapy massage in improving quality of life in patients with cancer* - research in process, 1999.

Wilkinson, S., Does aromatherapy enhance the quality of life of patients with advanced cancer. *Psycho Oncology*, 1995; 4(2):98-99.